C. Neal Ellis

Editor

Inherited Cancer Syndromes

Current Clinical Management

Second Edition

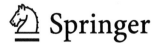 Springer

Editor
C. Neal Ellis
Professor of Surgery
Department of Surgery
University of South Alabama Medical Center
Mobile, AL 36617
USA
nellis@usouthal.ed

ISBN 978-1-4419-6820-3   e-ISBN 978-1-4419-6821-0
DOI 10.1007/978-1-4419-6821-0
Springer New York Dordrecht Heidelberg London

Library of Congress Control Number: 2010938363

Printed on acid-free paper

Springer is part of Springer Science+Business Media (www.springer.com)

Contents

Contributors

Kathryn R. Brown, MD
Department of Obstetrics, Gynecology and Women's Health, University
of Louisville Hospital, Louisville, KY 40202, USA

W. Donald Buie, MD, MSc, FRCS(C), FACS
Department of Surgery, Division of General Surgery, University of Calgary,
Calgary, Canada; 1403 29th St., NW Calgary, Alberta Canada T3H 1L8

James M. Church, MD, ChB, FRACS
Department of Colorectal Neoplasia, Sanford R. Weiss Center for Hereditary
Colorectal Cancer, Cleveland Clinic Foundation, Cleveland, OH 44195, USA

Charles E. Cox, MD, FACS
McCann Foundation Endowed Professor of Breast Surgery, Director, Breast
Health Clinical and Research Integrated Strategic Program (CRISP), USF Health
Department of Surgery, Carol and Frank Morsani Center for Advanced Health
Care, Tampa, FL 33612, USA

C. Neal Ellis, MD
Division of Colon and Rectal Surgery, West Penn Allegheny Health System,
PA 15212, Pittsburgh

Jeffrey M. Farma, MD
Assistant Professor of Surgery, Department of Surgical Oncology, Fox Chase
Cancer Center, Philadelphia, PA 19111, USA

Roy E. Gandy, MD
Department of Surgery, University of South Alabama Medical Center,
Mobile, AL 36617, USA

Ramona Hagmaier, MHS, PA-C
Physician Assistant, Skin Perfection Medical Spa, Mobile, AL 36695, USA

William J. Harb, MD
Baptist Hospital, Nashville, TN, USA
and
Cumberland Surgical Associates, PLC 2011 Church St. Suite 703, Nashville, TN
37203, USA

Brandie Heald, MS, CGC
Genomic Medicine Institute and the Sanford R. Weiss Center for Hereditary
Colorectal Neoplasio, Cleveland Clinic Foundation, Cleveland, OH 44195, USA

Anthony R. MacLean, MD, FRCS(C), FACS
Clinical Associate Professor of Surgery, Department of Surgery; Program
Director, Division of General Surgery, University of Calgary, Calgary, AB,
Canada

Deborah A. Nagle, MD
Division of Colon and Rectal Surgery, Beth Israel Deaconess Medical Center,
Harvard University, Boston, MA 02215, USA

Lynn P. Parker, MD
Director, Gynecology, Department of Obstetrics, Gynecology and Women's
Health, University of Louisville Hospital, Louisville, KY 40202, USA

Vitaliy Poylin, MD
Department of Surgery, Beth Israel Deaconess Medical Center/Harvard University
School of Medicine, Boston, MA 02215, USA

Adam I. Riker, MD
Oshsner Cancer Institute, Department of Surgery, 1514 Jefferson, New Orleans,
LA, USA

Charles B. Rodning, MD, PhD
Professor, Department of Surgery, University of South Alabama Medical Center,
Mobile, AL 36617, USA

Alfredo A. Santillan, MD, MPH
Division of Surgical Oncology, Department of Surgery, Cancer Therapy and
Research Center, University of Texas Health Science Center at San Antonio,
78229 San Antonio, TX, USA

Chapter 1
Obtaining and Using Genetic Information

C. Neal Ellis

Introduction

Our current understanding of the molecular pathophysiology of cancer explains many of the important epidemiology and clinical observations that have been made in the last 100 years. For example, the identification and characterization of genes responsible for hereditary cancer syndromes have explained the predisposition of members of affected families to develop site-specific cancer at a relatively young age [1]. A positive family medical history is now a leading risk factor for the subsequent development of many diseases including diabetes, neurologic disorders such as Huntington's chorea, atherosclerotic coronary vascular disease and many cancers including breast, ovarian, colon, and prostate cancer and melanoma [1–6]. The understanding of the molecular basis of cancer has been evolving rapidly since the completion of the Human Genome project. Several specific gene mutations have been implicated in predisposing patients to a variety of hereditary cancer syndromes [7–17]. This understanding has provided the ability to use genetic testing to estimate the risk, predict onset, and aid in assessing the prognosis of many forms of cancer. However, these genetic tests have also created complex issues and controversies regarding the use of the information obtained. The appropriate interpretation of test results with the implications for screening, preventive interventions, or clinical management decisions are not yet fully defined.

Cancer control efforts to reduce the incidence of cancer have focused primarily on prevention and early detection. These efforts will be most beneficial for individuals who are at highest risk. Thus, it is imperative that healthcare providers become familiar with the tools to assess a person's genetic risk of cancer, the general benefits and limitations of genetic testing in medical practice, and the process of making informed decisions about diagnosis and treatment of malignant disorders. The objective of this chapter is to generate a practical guide to aid physicians

C.N. Ellis (✉)
Division of Colon and Rectal Surgery, West Penn Allegheny Health System,
PA, 15212, Pittsburgh
e-mail: nellis@usouthal.edu

C.N. Ellis (ed.), *Inherited Cancer Syndromes: Current Clinical Management*,
DOI 10.1007/978-1-4419-6821-0_1, © Springer Science+Business Media, LLC 2011

in the assessment of the genetic risk of their patients for the development of cancer. The most prevalent inherited cancer syndromes are covered later in this book. The clinical scenarios presented in this chapter were selected to illustrate the strengths and weaknesses of current cancer genetic knowledge. This information is aimed toward providing the basic information a physician may need to identify those patients at high risk of developing cancer and assist in determining the need for further assessment, enhanced screening, preventive intervention, or referral. Several guidelines have been published at http://www.guidelines.gov that should further aid physicians in incorporating genetic risk assessment into their practices and are discussed in the chapters on the various diseases.

Collecting Family History of Cancer Information

The assessment of a patient for risk of cancer requires that the physician determine if one or more cancers are clustering in the patient's family and whether one is dealing with sporadic, familial, or inherited cases. This is complicated in that common cancers occur commonly. Thus, in a large family one might expect to see one or more cases of the more prevalent cancers. Many factors can lead to familial clustering of cancer such as chance, common environmental exposures and lifestyle, or the inheritance of mutated genes. The challenge in assessing a family cancer history is to determine which of these possibilities explains the cancers in a family. For example, if one is dealing with a shared environmental exposure such as tobacco smoke, education and smoking cessation programs would be appropriate. On the other hand, if an inherited gene mutation is suspected, management options would include aggressive cancer screening, and possibly prophylactic interventions such as surgery.

An essential step in identifying patients at high risk for hereditary cancer syndromes is to obtain a detailed family medical history for cancer [18]. Many physicians do not obtain a sufficiently detailed family history of cancer to identify a hereditary cancer syndrome. Moreover, it is not uncommon for healthcare providers to misinterpret or fail to act on the information provided [19–24]. Although patients are becoming more knowledgeable about their medical conditions, many will not present to their healthcare provider knowing they are a member of a family carrying a gene that predisposes them to cancer. It is the responsibility of the healthcare provider to identify patients who are members of families with high-risk hereditary cancer syndromes. The majority of the hereditary cancer syndromes include different types of cancers often affecting multiple generations. In general, the risk that a patient is a member of a high-risk hereditary cancer syndrome family increases as the number of generations and individuals with cancer increases and the age of the affected individuals decreases. One of the hallmarks of hereditary cancer is early age of onset. A history of cancers that appear in family members under the age of 50 should alert the clinician that they could be dealing with an inherited cancer syndrome.

Gleaning the necessary information requires a structured approach to obtaining a family medical history of cancer. The essential components of a family cancer

Table 1.1 Components of a
complete family cancer history

At least three generations
Ethnic background
For affected individuals
Type and site of primary cancer
Age at diagnosis of each primary cancer
Treatment facility/location
Occupational/environmental exposures
Age at death/current age

history are shown in Table 1.1. While there are several methods in which the information can be obtained, the most common method is to obtain the family cancer history at the time of the initial office encounter. However, patients rarely recall the detailed information necessary to adequately assess the possibility of an inherited cancer syndrome. A two-step process provides the most accurate information. During the initial office visit, a brief family history of cancer is obtained and the need to obtain more detailed information is explained. A structured family cancer history questionnaire is given to the patient to complete after discussion with other family members. This provides the patient the opportunity to contact family members and check medical or death records, which increases the completeness and accuracy of the information obtained. The questionnaire is subsequently returned to the healthcare provider. The validity of the aforementioned approaches to collecting a family medical history of cancer and the accuracy of the information reported by patients appear to be good [25–31]. In one study, 83% of patients correctly identified the primary cancer site in their first-degree relatives [26]. The reporting site was accurate in 67% of second-degree relatives and 60% of third-degree relatives. False positives were 5%. In another study, the accuracy of cancer reported in first- and second-degree relatives was 91% and 74%, respectively [27]. A mistake in identifying the presence or site of the cancer was found in only 4% of first-degree and 15% of second-degree relatives. Although a small amount of over-reporting by breast cancer patients of breast cancer in their families has been observed, the accuracy of reporting in first-degree relatives was 90% [29]. The false-negative reporting has been observed to vary by tumor site and to be greater in men, individuals of non-white race and older age. Other variables influencing false-negative reporting include time since cancer diagnosis, number of previous tumors, and type of treatment received [31]. The false-negative reporting rate for breast, colon, and prostate and bladder cancer was 20.8%, 42.1%, and 61.5%, respectively.

Another important aspect of the family cancer history which is frequently overlooked is the need to periodically repeat the process and update the pedigree. In our center, the family cancer history is updated at the time of each screening mammogram or colonoscopy for patients with a high risk of these malignancies based on their initial family history of cancer. It is not uncommon for a family with a suspicious but nondiagnostic family cancer history initially to progress to one that is diagnostic of a known hereditary cancer syndrome as family members age and additional members are added.

While it is recognized that the best estimate of an individual's cancer risk will depend on the accuracy and detail of the family cancer history, there will be situations where this will not be feasible. Adoption, small families, estrangement and many other situations could create a situation where the physician is unable to adequately assess the risk of an inherited cancer syndrome and make recommendations regarding genetic testing or some of the more invasive preventive interventions.

The next step in the process of genetic cancer risk assessment is to use the family history of cancer to construct a pedigree. Although one can hand draw the pedigree, there are several commercially available software programs and some in the public domain to aid in this process [32–35]. The pedigree should include all cancers, ages of diagnosis, and ages at death. It has been found to be useful to send the constructed pedigree back to the patient, asking them to confirm the accuracy of the information. It is not uncommon for the initial pedigree to be returned with corrections or additions. These changes are indicative of the visual aspect of the pedigree, the queries, and the additional time to think about their family cancer history which stimulates patients to refine the information. The detailed family history of cancer information obtained can now be used to assess a patient's risk of cancer and determine if the pedigree suggests a hereditary cancer syndrome.

Genetic Counseling

The initial management of any patient with a suspected inherited cancer syndrome is genetic counseling. Genetic counseling can be performed by the physician or a trained genetic counselor. Genetic counseling is a multi-step process which includes resolution of any ambiguities in the family cancer history and education about hereditary cancer syndromes and the implications of a hereditary disease for the patient's family. If indicated and desired, informed consent can be obtained and genetic testing performed. Informed consent for genetic testing should include discussion of genetic testing, including cost, benefits, limitations and risks, discussion of screening and management issues, discussion of employment and insurance issues and a review of the patient's concerns and questions.

The role of genetic testing in the diagnosis of an inherited cancer syndrome is often misunderstood. It is critical to understand that the diagnosis of these syndromes is made on the basis of a patient's history and clinical examination and their family medical history. While the discovery of a genetic defect by genetic testing can provide valuable diagnostic and prognostic information for a patient and their family, the failure to identify an abnormality does not mean that one is not present and does not exclude the diagnosis of an inherited cancer syndrome. For the affected patient, determination of their specific genetic abnormality can provide helpful prognostic information. Even though attempts to correlate genotypic information with the phenotypic manifestations of the disease have not been completely successful, certain specific patterns can be discerned.

After the specific genetic mutation has been identified in an affected family member, genetic testing for that specific defect can be offered to other members of the family who are at risk for inheriting the defect. In this circumstance, discovery of the abnormality in a patient who has yet to exhibit the disease can indicate the need for early and frequent screening for the manifestations of the disease and the possibility of passing the defect to their offspring. A family member who can be conclusively proven not to have inherited the defect, which is associated with the increased risk of malignancy in their family, is at no greater risk of cancer than the general population and needs neither aggressive screening for cancer nor is there a potential for their children to inherit the defect.

Table 1.2 lists a number of hereditary cancer syndromes for which the mutated gene(s) have been identified and genetic tests are available to identify these mutations. The website http://www.genetests.org is a convenient source for laboratories that perform various genetic tests and clinics that specializes in genetic evaluation of patients and reviews of various genetic disorders.

Table 1.2 Hereditary cancer syndromes for which genetic tests are available

Syndrome	Associated malignancies	Mode of inheritance	Gene
Breast/ovarian	Breast, ovarian, prostate, pancreatic	Dominant	BRCA1 BRCA2
Cowden	Breast, ovarian, follicular of thyroid, colon	Dominant	PTEN
Li-Fraumeni	Breast, brain, soft-tissue sarcomas, osteosarcomas, leukemia, adrenocortical carcinomas	Dominant	p53
Familial polyposis	Colon, desmoids hepatoblastoma central nervous syndrome	Dominant	APC
HNPCC	Colon, endometrial, ovarian, kidney, ureter, stomach, biliary tract, brain, small intestine	Dominant	MLH1 MSH2 MSH6
MYH-associated polyposis	Colon	Recessive	MYH
Peutz-Jeghers	GI, breast	Dominant	STKII
Hereditary pancreatic melanoma	Pancreas, melanoma	Dominant	VP16
MEN2A	Medullary thyroid, pheochromocytomas, parathyroid adenomas	Dominant	RET
MEN2B	Medullary thyroid, pheochromocytomas, mucosal neuromas	Dominant	RET
Neurofibromatous 1	Neurofibrosarcomas, pheochromocytomas, optic gliomas	Dominant	NF1
Neurofibromatous 2	Bilateral acoustic neuroma, other tumors of nervous system	Dominant	NF2
Wilms' tumor	Nephroblastoma, hepatoblastoma, rhabdomyosarcoma, neuroblastoma	Dominant	WT1

Clinical Scenarios

Using a select number of case scenarios, examples of how a family cancer history can be used to estimate a patient's risk of cancer, diagnose a hereditary cancer syndrome, and possibly refine the genetic risk through genetic testing will be presented. A pedigree analysis of an individual with a large family will often reveal one of the more prevalent cancers, e.g. breast or colon. However, the pattern of cancer may not fit the criteria for a hereditary cancer syndrome and may reflect the presence of sporadic cancer. Approximately 6–10% of breast and colon cancer cases are estimated to fit an autosomal dominant pattern of inheritance. A pedigree analysis is the only method to determine individuals who may be at high risk for cancer and would benefit from mutation testing.

Scenario 1: Breast Cancer

Figure 1.1 is the pedigree in which the family has a positive family history of breast cancer but the pattern does not meet any of the hereditary cancer syndrome criteria. The patient is a 41-year-old white female who was referred due to the presence of breast cancer in her mother and maternal aunt. The patient's mother developed unilateral breast cancer at age 36 years and a maternal aunt developed breast cancer at age 62 years. The maternal grandfather's sister developed breast cancer at an

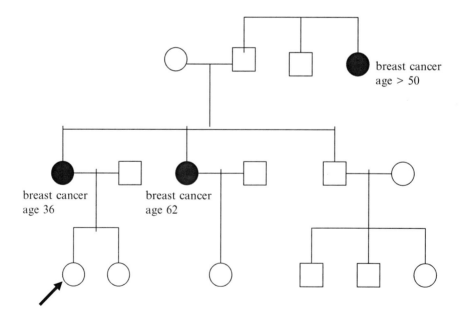

Fig. 1.1 Pedigree of a patient with nonfamilial breast cancer

unknown age, but it was believed to be above the age of 50. The referring physician was alerted by the appearance of breast cancer in the patient's mother below the age of 50, which is one of the hallmarks of hereditary breast cancer, and breast cancer in a maternal aunt and great aunt. However, the pattern of cancer in this family does not strongly suggest hereditary breast cancer.

There are models one can use to estimate the patient's risk of breast cancer. The Gail model uses age, age at menarche, age at first live birth, number of prior breast biopsies, and number of first-degree relatives affected with breast cancer to calculate the probability that a woman will develop breast cancer at various ages in life [36]. The National Cancer Institute distributes a software version of this model, which is available at http://cancertrials.nci.nih.gov/forms/CtRisk-Disk.html. Another breast cancer risk assessment tool is the Claus model, which estimates risk based solely on the number of maternal and paternal first- and second-degree relatives and the age at which they developed breast cancer [37]. In the original publication, a series of tables are provided that can be used to estimate risk based on various family history of cancer scenarios. A third model, the Bodian, can be used to estimate breast cancer risk for women in families where lobular neoplasia has been diagnosed [38]. Each of these models provides a reasonable estimate of risk for breast cancer for most women but has its limitations [39–41]. The Gail model does not take into account a family history of cancer. However, it has been reported to accurately assign a risk estimate for 87% of women [41]. The Gail and Claus models both fail to consider ovarian cancer risk, risk for women who have been diagnosed with lobular neoplasia, and the possibility of breast cancer predisposing gene mutations. The Gail model will overestimate the risk of women who do not carry a BRCA mutation and underestimate the risk in carriers of mutations [42]. For the patient in Fig. 1.1, the Gail model gave a lifetime probability of 19.9% that she would develop breast cancer compared to the population risk of 12.9%. This contrasts with the Claus model, which provided a probability of 29.6% that the patient would develop breast cancer by age 79. Approximately 19% of women who develop breast cancer have a positive family history [43, 44]. Of these, approximately 6–7% are due to mutations in either BRCA1 or BRCA2 [45–47]. One can determine the probability of BRCA1 or BRCA2 mutations occurring in a given family by use of the data obtained by Myriad Genetics Laboratories on 10,000 individuals who were referred to them for testing [48]. Myriad provides BRCA1 and BRCA2 mutation prevalence data in tabular form at http://www.myriad.com/med/brac/mutptables.htm. Using these data, the prevalence of deleterious mutations in BRCA1 and BRCA2 that have been observed in families with a history of cancer similar to the family in Fig. 1.1 is 4.4%. This estimate is based on the observation that the patient has not presented with breast or ovarian cancer, that of the two relatives who presented with breast cancer, only one occurred below the age of 50, and that no history of ovarian cancer at any age had been observed in any relative at the time of analysis. BRCAPRO is a family history model that uses Bayes theorem to calculate an individual's probability of developing breast cancer [49]. This model incorporates the probability that an individual carries a mutation in BRCA1 or BRCA2. The software program CancerGene calculates breast cancer risks using Gail, Claus, BRCAPRO, and Bodian models and is available at http://www3.utsouthwestern.edu/cancergene [50]. The software also draws a pedigree and calculates BRCA gene mutation probabilities. BRCAPRO has been shown to be better in discriminating between BRCA gene mutation carriers vs BRCA gene mutation noncarriers than cancer risk counselors [50]. Using the BRCAPRO model to estimate risk for the patient in Fig. 1.1 gave a risk of developing breast and ovarian cancer by age 86 of 12.3% and 1.8%, respectively. The probability that breast cancer in the patient's family was due to a BRCA1 or BRCA2 mutation using the BRCAPRO model was 2.2%, slightly less than the 4.4% derived from the Myriad tables [48]. Established guidelines have recommended that BRCA genetic testing be considered for individuals whose family history of breast/ovarian cancer suggested an estimated prior probability of a BRCA mutation greater than 10%. Additional guidelines have stipulated that testing should only be offered when the test can be adequately interpreted and the results will influence medical management. Thus the probability that breast cancer in the patient's family in Fig. 1.1 is due to a deleterious mutation in one of the breast cancer susceptibility genes is sufficiently low that testing for BRCA mutations is not indicated.

Take Home Message

There are a number of models, especially for breast cancer, available to assist clinicians in determining who would benefit from genetic testing.

Scenario 2: Breast Cancer

Figure 1.2 is the pedigree of a 24-year-old female who is concerned about her risk of breast cancer. Although her father carries no cancer diagnosis, two of his three sisters were diagnosed with premenopausal breast cancer, and his mother was affected with breast and ovarian cancer before age 45. According to the Myriad model, the patient

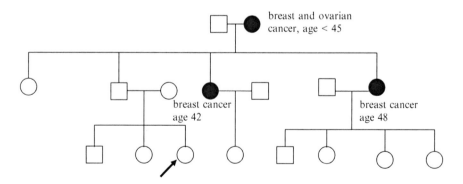

Fig. 1.2 Pedigree of a patient with Hereditary Breast/Ovarian Cancer syndrome

has a 16.4% risk for carrying a deleterious mutation in either *BRCA1* or *BRCA2*. Her risk of breast cancer as predicted by the Claus model is 0.6% by age 59, 2.0% by age 39, 5.2% by age 49, 9.8% by age 59, 14.7% by age 69, and 18.4% by age 79. The limitations of the models are discussed, and the patient is counseled about her Mendelian risk if a *BRCA1* or *BRCA2* has caused the cancers in her family: specifically her father has a 50% risk of having inherited the mutation from his mother, while the patient's risk is 25%. She is further counseled that, if she has the mutation, her risk for breast cancer is approximately 85%, while her risk of ovarian cancer is 16–60%. Her risk for pancreatic cancer may also be increased. The benefits, limitations, and risks of genetic testing are reviewed, and the benefit of first testing her living affected aunt is discussed. Screening recommendations based on her family history alone are reviewed. She is also guided through different scenarios regarding her possible mutation status and how screening and management recommendations may be influenced based on her genetic status. She expresses her interest in testing, as well as her concerns over the risks to her young daughter when she is older. The initial counseling session ends when the patient decides to contact her aunt regarding her willingness to pursue genetic counseling and testing. The aunt is subsequently tested and learns she carries a deleterious mutation in *BRCA1*. The patient returns for testing, and at her results disclosure session 3 weeks later she learns that she does not carry the mutation. Her risk for breast and ovarian cancer is no greater than that of the general population, and appropriate screening recommendations are made. It is important to understand that if the aunt had not agreed to testing, the negative test result in this patient would have been less informative. Although no mutation was found in *BRCA1* and *BRCA2*, the possibility of another gene being responsible for the cancers in her family would not have been ruled out, and her screening recommendations would have reflected her family history. She would have been assigned to the high-risk category, although this patient learned that she has not inherited the cancer susceptibility mutation that has caused the cancer in her family, her paternal cousins are at risk for the identified genetic mutation. After learning about her risk, a female cousin undergoes testing and learns she is positive for the mutation. She is anxious over her heightened risks and meets with a surgeon to discuss prophylactic mastectomy and oophorectomy. She decides that she will follow the recommended high-risk screening procedures until she has completed childrearing; at which time she may consider prophylactic mastectomy and/or oophorectomy.

Take Home Message

There are a number of points in this scenario:

1. Genetic testing of a known affected family member, if at all possible, provides the best opportunity to obtain clinically useful information.
2. If a patient can be *conclusively* proven to not have the known defect in their family, they have no greater risk of cancer than the general population and do not need aggressive screening or prophylactic surgery.

3. Once the specific defect in a family is known, at-risk family members after genetic counseling and informed consent can be tested for that specific defect at much less cost.

Scenario 3: Breast Cancer

Figure 1.3 is the pedigree of a family where the patient presented with endometrial cancer at age 37 but had a significant family history of breast/ovarian cancer. One of the patient's sisters developed breast cancer at ages 48 and 53, and another sister developed bilateral breast cancer at age 40. The patient's mother was diagnosed with ovarian cancer at age 39 and breast cancer at age 62. Her maternal grandmother developed bilateral breast cancer at age 52. Her paternal grandmother had developed ovarian and cervical cancer, but age at onset was unknown. The pattern certainly fits the criteria for Hereditary Breast/Ovarian Cancer syndrome, e.g. breast cancer onset below the age of 50, bilateral breast cancer, and ovarian cancer at any age. The probability of a deleterious *BRCA* mutation in this family was 16.5% by BRCAPRO and 16.4% by the Myriad tables. However, on genetic testing, the patient did not possess a *BRCA1* or *BRCA2* deleterious mutation. The dilemma in counseling this patient is that one cannot predict if her risk for developing another breast cancer or ovarian cancer or the risk to her children is elevated over the risk estimate based on family history alone. This is a family where their cancers may be due to the approximately 5% of mutated genes that are responsible for Hereditary Breast/Ovarian Cancer that have yet to be defined. For this patient, it cannot be conclusively proven that she did not inherit a genetic defect which can lead to breast cancer. Therefore, most would recommend this patient and her family should undergo the same aggressive screening for breast and ovarian cancer that would be recommended for patients with a known *BRCA* mutation.

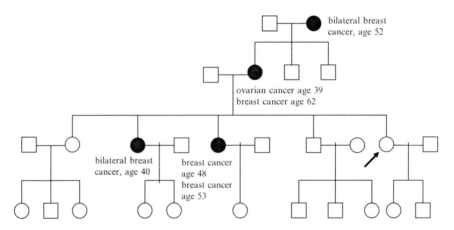

Fig. 1.3 Pedigree of a patient with Hereditary Breast/Ovarian Cancer syndrome

Take Home Message

In a family who obviously has a familial cancer syndrome on evaluation of their pedigree; failure to identify a defect with genetic testing does not mean that the family does not have a defect. Instead this should be interpreted as the family's hereditary cancer syndrome being related to some other, as yet unidentified, genetic defect.

Scenario 4: Breast Cancer

Approximately 1 in 40 individuals of Ashkenazi Jewish descent carry one of the following so-called "founder mutations": 185delAG or 5382insC in BRCA1 or 6174delT in BRCA2 [51–54]. It has been suggested that Ashkenazi Jewish women consider testing for these mutations if they have developed early-onset breast or ovarian cancer at any age regardless of their family history of cancer. Figure 1.4 is the pedigree of a family of Ashkenazi Jewish descent where six sisters developed breast cancer. However, none of the sisters developed breast cancer before the age of 60. The patient was concerned about the risk to her daughter and therefore requested testing for the Ashkenazi Jewish panel of BRCA1 and BRCA2 mutations. The probability that breast cancer in this family was due to BRCA mutations based on the Myriad tables and BRCAPRO model was 3.2% and 77.2%, respectively. The patient did not test positive for any of these founder mutations. A comprehensive BRCA analysis for this family is indicated since other predisposing mutations have been reported in individuals of Ashkenazi Jewish descent [55, 56].

Take Home Message

Genetic defects can be ethnic specific and can be tested for separately.

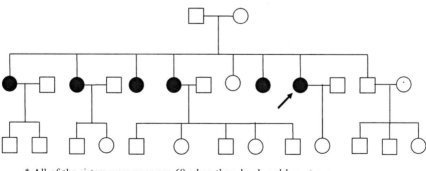

* All of the sisters were over age 60 when they developed breast cancer.

Fig. 1.4 Pedigree of an Ashkenazi Jewish family with familial breast cancer

Scenario 5: Colorectal Cancer

Colorectal cancer is the second leading cause of death by cancer in the United States. While approximately 75–80% of colorectal cancer is sporadic, it is estimated that 20–25% of cases are familial, and 6–10% of cases are due to familial adenomatous polyposis (FAP) or hereditary nonpolyposis colorectal cancer (HNPCC) [15, 57–60]. A person with a first-degree relative who developed colorectal cancer has a 2% risk by age 50 and 7% by age 70 of developing colorectal cancer [58]. The risk estimate will vary depending on the affected relative (parents or sibling) and the site of the cancer. This risk estimate will be greater for a family with a hereditary colorectal cancer syndrome [59].

Figure 1.5 is the pedigree of a 16-year-old male who is brought for evaluation of rectal bleeding by his mother. His mother has FAP diagnosed at age 32 when she developed a colon cancer. His maternal grandmother and uncle died of colorectal cancer at age 42 and 48 years, respectively. He has one maternal cousin who had had a colectomy for FAP. FAP is a dominantly inherited colorectal cancer syndrome that accounts for about 1% of colorectal cancers. It is caused by a mutation of the *APC* gene and is characterized clinically by the hundreds to thousands of colonic adenomas that develop at an early age. Patients with FAP may also develop a variety of extracolonic manifestations including gastroduodenal neoplasia, desmoid tumors, and osteomas.

The patient was counseled about the known FAP in his family, and his risks are discussed. He is counseled about his 50% risk for having inherited the FAP mutation from his mother, and his cancer risks are reviewed. Genetic testing was discussed as it could provide some prognostic information. The initial counseling session comes to an end, and the patient agrees to undergo screening colonoscopy. At colonoscopy, the patient is found to have over 50 adenomatous polyps. Colectomy is recommended and screening recommendations are made based on his risk of developing extracolonic manifestations of FAP.

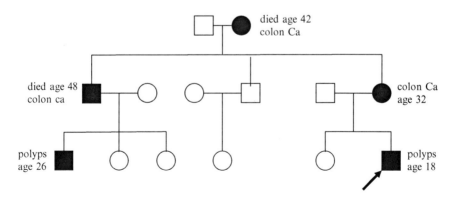

Fig. 1.5 Pedigree of a patient with FAP

Take Home Message

The onset of FAP frequently occurs before patients are of age to give consent. Except in special circumstances, genetic testing for cancer genes is not recommended for those unable to give consent.

Scenario 6: Colorectal Cancer

Figure 1.6 is the pedigree of a 48-year-old man who underwent colonoscopy for the evaluation of rectal bleeding. At colonoscopy, the patient was found to have 38 adenomatous polyps. On evaluation of the family cancer history however, while his sister was found to have 24 polyps at age 44 years, there is no evidence of colorectal pathology in the previous generations. In approximately 10% of patients with polyposis, the family cancer history will show no evidence to suggest a dominantly inherited colorectal cancer syndrome. Possible explanations for this include a new mutation, or questions of paternity, adoption, or denial.

The patient was counseled about the clinical diagnosis of FAP, and his risks for extracolonic manifestations are discussed. He is counseled about his 50% risk for passing the FAP mutation to his children. Genetic testing was discussed because it could provide some prognostic information. The initial counseling session comes to an end, and the patient agrees to undergo genetic testing.

He returns and is informed that genetic testing revealed no germline abnormality of the *APC* gene. Another possibility in this patient is *MYH*-associated polyposis. It is usually impossible to distinguish polyposis related to bi-allelic *MYH* mutations from FAP clinically in an individual patient. On evaluation of the family medical history however, the distinction is usually obvious. While FAP has an autosomal dominant pattern of inheritance, *MYH*-associated polyposis is inherited in an autosomal recessive

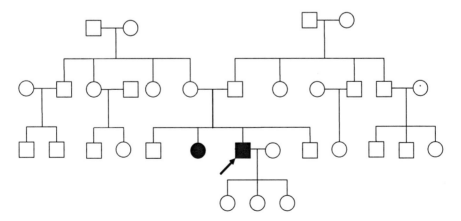

Fig. 1.6 Pedigree of a patient with *MYH*-associated polyposis

manner requiring the defect to be present on both sides of the family. The number of polyps in MAP is variable, having a reported range of 5–750, with a median of approximately 50 polyps, and 36% of patients having over 100 polyps [61, 62]. Colorectal cancer occurs in approximately 50% of patients at a mean age of 50 years with a range of 30–65 years. The cancers are usually left-sided, with multiple colorectal cancers present in 24% of the patients at diagnosis [62]. Extracolonic manifestations have also been associated with bi-allelic *MYH* mutations and include two reported cases of gastric cancer (one at 17 years of age) and two cases of duodenal polyps. Congenital hypertrophy of the retinal pigment epithelium and osteomas have also been reported [62–64].

The patient undergoes testing for a *MYH* mutation and is found to have a bi-allelic defect. Colectomy is recommended and screening recommendations are made based on his risk of developing extracolonic manifestations of FAP. The patient is also counseled that his children have a 50% risk of inheriting the defect but that this is of no known clinical significance unless they also inherited a *MYH* mutation from their mother.

Take Home Message

MYH-associated polyposis is the first inherited cancer syndrome to be identified which has a recessive mode of inheritance but will likely not be the last. For patients with these recessive syndromes, the concern is more for their siblings than for other members of the family.

Scenario 7: Colon Cancer

Hereditary Nonpolyposis Colon Cancer (HNPCC or Lynch syndrome) is a hereditary cancer syndrome that requires a detailed family cancer history to diagnose the disorder and determine if family members would benefit from mutation testing. This is an autosomal dominant inherited disorder that accounts for approximately 6% of all colorectal cancer and is the most common inherited colorectal cancer syndrome. This syndrome has been defined by several criteria. The most stringent is the Amsterdam criteria, which requires three relatives, one of whom is a first-degree relative of the other two, diagnosed with colorectal cancer in two generations, with one or more cases diagnosed before the age of 50 and FAP had been excluded [65]. The Modified Amsterdam [66] and Amsterdam II [67] include cancer at several extracolonic sites including the endometrium, ovary, stomach, small bowel, hepatobiliary tract, pancreas, ureter, renal pelvis, and breast [68, 69].

Hereditary nonpolyposis colon cancer is due to mutations that occur in several mismatch repair (MMR) genes, although most testing is limited to MSH2, MLH1 and MSH6, where the majority of the HNPCC predisposing mutations occur [70]. Microsatellite instability is the hallmark of mismatch repair deficiency.

Microsatellites are mono-, di-, and trinucleotides repeats which are scattered throughout the genome, and due to their repetitive nature are prone to errors during replication [65–67, 71, 72]. MMR deficiency leads to an increased susceptibility to tumor formation [68, 69]. Microsatellite instability is present in all HNPCC colorectal cancers; it also occurs in 15% of sporadic colorectal tumors [69, 70, 73, 74]. The Bethesda Guidelines were designed to help determine which patients should be tested for microsatellite instability (MSI) [73]. Of all the clinical criteria available, the Bethesda Guidelines have been reported as the most sensitive for detecting HNPCC, but they are less specific [75]. The cost-effectiveness of genetic testing is increased if one can screen the tumor of a family member for MSI prior to testing [76].

Another option for screening tumors for deficiencies of the mismatch repair genes prior to genetic testing is immunohistochemical staining. Immunohistochemical stains for *MLH1*, *MSH2*, and *MSH6* are available. Immunohistochemical staining is not 100% specific for HNPCC because 10–15% of sporadic cancers can have and acquired inactivation of *MLH1* by hypermethylation of the *MLH1* promoter region [70, 73–75].

Figure 1.7 is the pedigree of a 30-year-old male seeking information about his risk for colon cancer. A paternal aunt and uncle, his grandmother, and a great aunt all presented with cancers consistent with HNPCC. His father had eight adenomatous polyps detected on examination at age 53 and elected to have a colectomy. He has two paternal cousins with adenomatous colon polyps before the age of 40. The patient was counseled about the strong suspicion of HNPCC in his family, and his risks are discussed. He is counseled about his 50% risk for having inherited an HNPCC mutation from his father, and his cancer risks are reviewed. He reveals that his sister is estranged from the family, and he has not spoken to her in a number of years. He does not know if he can or is willing to contact her about her own risks. Screening for deficiencies of mismatch repair by MSI testing and immunohistochemical staining are not an option for this patient because no tumor tissue was

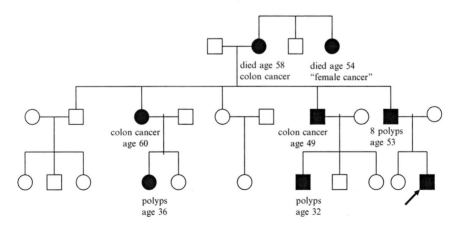

Fig. 1.7 Pedigree of a patient with HNPCC

available for these studies. Genetic testing is discussed and the utility of testing his uncle first is explained. The initial counseling session comes to an end, and the patient contacts his uncle during the following week to assess his willingness to pursue genetic testing. His uncle declines genetic testing but his father consents and is found to have a deleterious mutation in *MLH1*. The patient decides to proceed with testing and returns 3 weeks later and learns that he also has the *MLH1* mutation. Screening recommendations are made based on his high risk of developing colorectal cancer. His sister's risks for uterine and colorectal cancer are also discussed, and he decides that he will try to locate her to inform her of the risks. He also decides to notify other family members of the potential for them to have inherited the genetic defect.

Take Home Message

This patient's uncle's refusal to undergo genetic testing significantly decreased the likelihood of obtaining useful information in this situation. Many would question the cost effectiveness of performing genetic testing on this patient's father since he is not clearly affected by the disease.

Scenario 8: Colon Cancer

Figure 1.8 is a pedigree of a 36-year-old white female who was recently diagnosed with colon cancer. Her father died of colorectal cancer at age 48, and a paternal uncle had colorectal cancer at age 35. Her paternal grandmother was diagnosed with colon and breast cancer at ages 50 and 53, respectively. The patient was counseled about the strong suspicion of HNPCC in her family, and her risks were discussed. She is counseled about her 50% risk for having inherited mutation of the

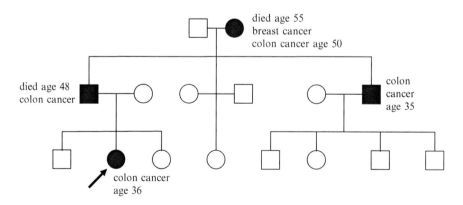

Fig. 1.8 Pedigree of a family with Familial Colorectal Cancer Syndrome Type X

mismatch repair genes. MSI testing and immunohistochemical staining are discussed as screening tests for deficiencies of mismatch repair prior to genetic testing. The patient agrees to MSI staining and immunohistochemical staining of her tumor. The patient returns 3 weeks later and is informed that her cancer does not have microsatellite instability and that immunohistochemical staining show no defects in *MLH1, MSH2,* or *MSH6*.

Recently, an article in the *Journal of the American Medical Association* separated a group of Amsterdam Criteria-positive families according to whether their tumors showed microsatellite instability or not [77]. Approximately 455 of the families did show microsatellite instability, conclusive evidence of a mismatch repair defect, and of the diagnosis of HNPCC. The remaining families had microsatellite stable tumors and are therefore not HNPCC. These families were classified as "familial colorectal cancer syndrome type X." The cancer risk in Syndrome X families was for colorectal cancer alone, and was about one-third that seen in HNPCC.

Since her cancer did not have microsatellite instability, this patient was considered to have familial colorectal cancer syndrome type X. While the risk of this patient developing a subsequent colorectal cancer, and her family's risk of developing colorectal cancer is not as high as those with HNPCC, they are still much greater than the risk of the general population and the screening recommendations are made based on their high risk of developing colorectal cancer. However, she is counseled that her risks for uterine cancer or the other extracolonic manifestations of HNPCC are no greater than the general population.

Take Home Message

The diagnosis of an inherited cancer syndrome is made on the basis of a patient's family history of cancer. If the specific defect cannot be found, then at-risk family members should be considered to have the syndrome and the same aggressive screening as would be performed for patients with known defects should be recommended.

Conclusions

Assessing a patients' genetic risk of cancer is a complex undertaking. Assessing cancer genetic risk is a multi-step process that intimately involves the patient in obtaining information of their family. After a family risk of cancer information is obtained and a risk estimate is generated, genetic counseling is required. The counseling session should not only cover the genetic features of the disorder and the estimated risk for the patient and other family members but should also cover the appropriate genetic testing, cancer screening programs, and preventive interventions that might be considered. It should be recognized by the healthcare provider that a family's history of cancer is not static. Therefore, the patient should be informed that his or her risk and the risk of family members might change should additional cases of cancer appear in the family.

As was illustrated by the cases presented, there is still a void in our knowledge of hereditary cancer. However, the knowledge is increasing exponentially. In the future, healthcare providers will have the tools to more accurately predict the development of a cancer. This genetic revolution has captured the imagination of the public. More and more patients are becoming aware of their family history of disease and asking their physician about the impact of this information on their health. Thus, healthcare providers are being increasingly challenged by their patients to stay abreast of these advances.

References

1. Lynch HT, Lynch JF. Familial factors and genetic predisposition to cancer: Population studies. Cancer Detect Prev 1991;15:49–57.
2. Woolf CM. An investigation of the familial aspects of carcinoma of the prostate. Cancer 1960;13:739.
3. Anderson DE. Some characteristics of familial breast cancer. Cancer 1971;28:1500–1504.
4. Easton D, Petro J. The contribution of inherited predisposition to cancer incidence. Cancer Surv 1990;9:395–416.
5. Ahnen DJ. Genetics of colon cancer. West J Med 1991;154:700–705.
6. Offit K, Brown K. Quantitating familial cancer risks: A resource for clinical oncologists. J Clin Oncol 1994;12:1724–1736.
7. Perera FP. Molecular epidemiology: Insights into cancer susceptibility, risk assessment, and prevention. JNCI 1996;88:496–509.
8. Li FP, Garber JE, Friend SH, et al. Recommendations on predictive testing for germ line p53 mutations among cancer-prone individuals. JNCI 1992;84:1156–1160.
9. Berchuck A, Cirisano F, Lancaster JM, et al. Role of BRCA1 mutation screening in the management of familial ovarian cancer. Am J Obstet Gynecol 1996;175:738–746.
10. Pasini B, Ceccherini I, Romeo G. RET mutations in human disease. Trends Genet 1996;12:138–144.
11. Fearon ER. Human cancer syndromes: Clues to the origin and nature of cancer. Science 1997;278:1043–1050.
12. Lindor NM, Greene MH. The concise handbook of family cancer syndromes. JNCI 1998;90:1039–1071.
13. Eng C, Hampel H, de la Chapelle A. Genetic testing for cancer predisposition. Ann Med 2000;52:371–400.
14. Couch V, Lindor NM, Karnes PS, et al. Von Hippel-Lindau disease. Mayo Clin Proc 2000;75:265–272.
15. Giardiello FM, Brensinger JD, Petersen GM. AGA technical review on hereditary colorectal cancer and genetic testing. Gastroenterology 2001;121:198–213.
16. Bratt O. Hereditary prostate cancer: Clinical aspects. J Urol 2002;168:906–913.
17. Marsh D, Zori R. Genetic insights into familial cancers – update and recent discoveries. Cancer Lett 2002;26:125–164.
18. Lynch HT, Fusaro RM, Lynch JF. Family history of cancer. Ann NY Acad Sci 1995;768:12–29.
19. Lynch HT, Paulson J, Severin M, et al. Failure to diagnose hereditary colorectal cancer and its medicolegal implications. A hereditary nonpolyposis colorectal cancer case. Dis Colon Rectum 1999;42:31–35.

20. Acton RT, Burst NM, Casebeer L, et al. Knowledge, attitudes and behaviors of Alabama's primary care physicians regarding cancer genetics. Acad Med 2000;75:850–852.
21. Ruo L, Cellini C, La-Calle JP Jr, et al. Limitations of family cancer history assessment at initial consultation. Dis Colon Rectum 2001;44:98–104.
22. Lynch HT. Cancer family history and genetic testing: Are malpractice adjudications waiting to happen? Am J Gastroenterol 2002;97:518–520.
23. Bunn JY, Bosompra K, Ashikaga T, et al. Factors influencing intention to obtain a genetic test for colon cancer risk: A population-based study. Prev Med 2002;34:567–577.
24. Batra S, Valdimarsdottir H, McGovern M, et al. Awareness of genetic testing for colorectal cancer predisposition among specialists in gastroenterology. Am J Gastroenterol 2002;97:729–733.
25. Acton RT, Go RCP, Roseman JM, et al. Use of self-administered family history of disease instruments to predict individuals at risk for cardiovascular diseases, hypertension and diabetes. Am J Hum Genet 1989;45:A275.
26 Love R, Evans M, Josten DM. The accuracy of patient reports of a family history of cancer. J Chron Dis 1985;38:289–293.
27. Koch M, Gaedke H, Jenkins H. Family history of ovarian cancer patients: A case–control study. Int J Epidemiol 1989;18:782–785.
28. Bondy ML, Strom SS, Colopy MW, et al. Accuracy of family history of cancer obtained through interviews with relatives of patients with childhood sarcoma. J Clin Epidemiol 1994;47:89–96.
29. Parent ME, Ghadirian P, Lacroix A, et al. Accuracy of reports of familial breast cancer in a case-control series. Epidemiology 1995;6:184–186.
30. Aitken J, Bain C, Ward M, et al. How accurate is self-reported family history of colorectal cancer? Am J Epidemiol 1995;141:863–871.
31. Desai MM, Bruce ML, Desai RA, et al. Validity of self-reported cancer history: A comparison of health interview data and cancer registry records. Am J Epidemiol 2001;153:299–306.
32. Progeny pedigree drawing software. http://www.progeny2000.com.
33. Cyrillic pedigree drawing software. http://www.cyrillicsoftware.com.
34. FTREE. A family tree printing program for PC/DOS and compatibles and DEC VAX computers that use Hewlett-Packard laser jet compatible printers. epi2.soph.uab.edu.
35. Fil Quiaoit, Pedigree Data Processing SYStem (PDPSys). 1998. http://lynx.fhcrc.org/_qge/d.html/software/pdpsys.html.
36. Gail MH, Brinton LA, Byar DP, et al. Projecting individualized probabilities of developing breast cancer for white females who are being examined annually. JNCI 1989;81:1879–1886.
37. Claus EB, Risch N, Thompson WD. Autosomal dominant inheritance of early-onset breast cancer. Cancer 1994;73:643–651.
38. Bodian CA, Perzin KH, Lattes R. Lobular neoplasia: Long term risk of breast cancer and relation to other factors. Cancer 1996;78:1024–1034.
39. McGuigan KA, Ganz PA, Breant C. Agreement between breast cancer risk estimates. JNCI 1996;88:1315–1317.
40. McTiernan A, Gilligan MA, Redmond C. Assessing individual risk for breast cancer: Risky business. J Clin Epidemiol 1997;50:547–556.
41. Euhus DM, Leitch M, Huth JF, et al. Limitations of the Gail model in the specialized breast cancer risk assessment clinic. Breast J 2002;8:23–27.
42. Costantino JP, Gail MH, Pee D, et al. Validation studies for models projecting the risk of invasive and total breast cancer incidence. JNCI 1999;91:1541–1548.
43. Slattery MI, Kerber RA. A comprehensive evaluation of family history and breast cancer risk: The Utah Population Database. JAMA 1993;270:1563–1568.
44. Colditz GA, Willett WC, Hunter DJ, et al. Family history, age and risk of breast cancer: Prospective data from the Nurses' Health Study. JAMA 1993;270:338–343.
45. Couch FJ, DeShano ML, Blackwood A, et al. BRCA1 mutations in women attending clinics that evaluate the risk of breast cancer. N Engl J Med 1997;336:1409–1415.

46. Shattuck-Eidens D, Oliphant A, McClure M, et al. BRCA1 sequence analysis in women at high risk for susceptibility mutations. JAMA 1997;278:1242–1250.
47. Frank TS, Manley SA, Olopade OI, et al. Sequence analysis of BRCA 1 and BRCA 2: Correlation of mutations with family history and ovarian cancer risk. J Clin Oncol 1998;16:2417–2425.
48. Frank TS, Deffenbaugh AM, Reid JE, et al. Clinical characteristics of individuals with germline mutations in BRCA1 and BRCA2: Analysis of 10,000 individuals. J Clin Oncol 2002;20:1480–1490.
49. Euhus DM. Understanding mathematical models for breast cancer risk assessment and counseling. Breast J 2001;7:224–232.
50. Euhus DM, Smith KC, Robinson L, et al. Pretest prediction of BRCA1 or BRCA2 mutation by risk counselors and the computer model BRCAPRO. JNCI 2002;94:844–851.
51. Struewing JP, Hartge P, Wacholder S, et al. The risk of cancer associated with specific mutations of BRCA1 and BRCA2 among Ashkenazi Jews. N Engl J Med 1997;336:1401–1408.
52. Abeliovich D, Kaduri L, Lerer I, et al. The founder mutations 185delAG and 5382insC in BRCA1 and 6174delT in BRCA2 appear in 60% of ovarian cancer and 30% of early-onset breast cancer patients among Ashkenazi women. Am J Hum Genet 1997;60:505–514.
53. Warner E, Foulkes W, Goodwin P, et al. Prevalence and penetrance of BRCA1 and BRCA2 gene mutations in unselected Ashkenazi Jewish women with breast cancer. JNCI 1999;91:1241–1247.
54. Beller U, Halle D, Catane R, et al. High frequency of BRCA1 and BRCA2 germline mutations in Ashkenazi Jewish ovarian cancer patients, regardless of family history. Gynecol Oncol 1997;67:123–126.
55. Robson ME, Offit K. New BRCA2 mutation in an Ashkenazi Jewish family with breast and ovarian cancer. Lancet 1997;350:117–118.
56. Schubert EL, Lee MK, Mefford JE, et al. BRCA22 in American families with four or more cases of breast or ovarian cancer: Recurrent and novel mutations, variable expression, penetrance, and the possibility of families whose cancer is not attributable to BRCA1 or BRCA2. Am J Hum Genet 1997;60:1031–1040.
57. Terdiman JP, Conrad PG, Sleisenger MH. Genetic testing in hereditary colorectal cancer: Indications and procedures. J Gastroenterol 1999;94:2344–2356.
58. Johns LE, Kee F, Collins BJ, et al. Colorectal cancer mortality in first-degree relatives of early-onset colorectal cancer cases. Dis Colon Rectum 2002;45:681–686.
59. Ivanovich JL, Read TE, Ciske DJ, et al. A practical approach to familial and hereditary colorectal cancer. Am J Med 1999;107:68–77.
60. American Gastroenterological Association. Medical position statement: Hereditary colorectal cancer and genetic testing. Gastroenterology 2001;121:195–197.
61. Sampson JR, Dolwani S, Jones S, et al. Autosomal recessive colorectal polyposis due to inherited mutations of MYH. Lancet 2003;362:39–41.
62. Lipton L, Tomlinson I. The multiple colorectal adenoma phenotype and MYH, a base excision repair gene. Clin Gastroenterol Hepatol 2004;8:633–638.
63. Jones S, Emmerson P, Maynard J, et al. Biallelic germline mutations in MYH predispose to multiple colorectal adenomas and somatic G:C(right arrow)T:A mutations. Hum Mol Genet 2002;11:2961–2967.
64. Venesio T, Molatore S, Catteno F, et al. High frequency of MYH mutations in a subset of patients with familial adenomatous polyposis. Gastroenterology 2004;126:1681–1685.
65. Ionov Y, Peinado MA, Maikhosyan S, et al. Ubiquitous somatic mutations in simple repeated sequences reveal a new mechanism for colonic carcinogenesis. Nature 1993;363:558–561.
66. Saletti P, Edwin ID, Pack K, et al. Microsatellite instability: application in hereditary nonpolyposis colorectal cancer. Ann Oncol 2001;12:151–160.
67. Kuwada SK, Ncklason, Burt RW. Biology and molecular genetics. Colorectal cancer. Ed. Saltz LB. Humana Press, Totowa, NJ 2002;14.
68. Parsons R, Li GM, Longley MJ, et al. Hypermutability and mismatch repair deficiency in RER-cells. Cell 1993;75:1227–1236.

69. Hemminki A, Peltomaki P, Mecklin JP, et al. Loss of wild type MLH1 gene is a feature of hereditary nonpolyposis colorectal cancer. Nat Genet 1994;8:405–410.
70. Bubb VJ, Curtis LJ, Cunningham C, et al. MSI and the role of hMSH2 in sporadic colorectal cancer. Oncogene 1996;12:2641–2649.
71. Aaltonen LA, Peltomaki P, Leach FS, et al. Clues to the pathogenesis of familial colorectal cancer. Science 1993;260:812–816.
72. Thibodoeau SN, Bren G, Schaid D. MSI in cancer of the proximal colon. Science 1993; 260:816–819.
73. Borresen AL, Lothe RA, McLing GI, et al. Somatic mutations in the hMSH2 gene in microsatellite unstable colorectal carcinomas. Hum Mol Genet 1995;4:2065–2072.
74. Herman JG, Umar A, Polyak K, et al. Incidence and functional consequences of hMLI1 promoter hypermethylation in colorectal carcinoma. Proc Natl Acad Sci USA 1998;95:8698–8702.
75. Vasen HF, Mecklin JP, Kahn PM, Lynch HT. The International Collaborative Group on Hereditary Non-Polyposis Colorectal Cancer (ICG-HNPCC). Dis Colon Rectum 1991;34:424–425.
76. Park JG, Vasen HF, Park YJ, et al. Suspected HNPCC and Amsterdam critical II: evaluation of mutation detection rate, an international collaborative study. Int J Colorectal Dis 2002;17:109–114.
77. Lindor NM, Rabe K, Petersen GM, et al. Lower cancer incidence in Amsterdam-I criteria families without mismatch repair deficiency: familial colorectal cancer type X. JAMA 2005;293:1979–1985.

Chapter 2
Cancer and Genetic Counseling

Brandie Heald and James M. Church

Introduction

All cancer is genetic. Cancer is a disease caused by an accumulation of genetic damage that interferes with the regulation of cell growth, differentiation, and death. Most cancer-causing genetic damage is acquired either due to environmental exposures, carcinogens, or chance. This type of genetic damage is somatic and does not present a risk to offspring. Accordingly, the majority of cancers occur sporadically. However, some cancers are familial, occurring as a cluster of similar cancers that occur within a family more frequently than expected by chance. These cancers do not follow a clearly hereditary pattern; they are thought to arise from shared genetic and environmental factors. Individuals within these families are at increased risk of developing the type of cancer found in their relatives. Finally, it is estimated that 5–10% of cancers are hereditary, occurring because of transmission of a genetic mutation in the germline. Individuals in these families are usually at increased risk for more than one type of cancer. Identification of a hereditary cancer syndrome is critical to help patients and their families understand what their lifetime risk of cancer is, help them to cope with the emotional response of knowing this risk, and develop a plan for management of this risk. The hereditary nature of some cancers has many implications for patients and families, implications that have become increasingly complex as genetic technology has become more sophisticated. Evaluation of a family history, explanation of the genetics of hereditary cancer syndromes, facilitation of genetic testing and discussion of the results, and advising about genetic discrimination and family planning are beyond the scope of the family practitioner or medical specialist. These are the roles of the genetic counselor. The purpose of this chapter is to describe the place of genetic counseling in the

B. Heald (✉)
Genomic Medicine Institute and the Sanford R. Weiss Center for Hereditary Colorectal Neoplasio, Cleveland Clinic Foundation, Cleveland, OH 44195, USA
e-mail: leachb@ccf.org

C.N. Ellis (ed.), *Inherited Cancer Syndromes: Current Clinical Management*,
DOI 10.1007/978-1-4419-6821-0_2, © Springer Science+Business Media, LLC 2011

management of hereditary cancer, focusing on general principles that may be applied to all syndromes.

Background

A gene is a particular segment of DNA that carries the biochemical code for a particular protein. Genes are packed into chromosomes, which are organized into 22 pairs of autosomes and one pair of sex chromosomes. All chromosomes are housed in the cell's nucleus. Each person receives one copy of each chromosome from each parent and therefore one copy of each gene from each parent. There is a huge amount of variation within human DNA enabling the existence of billions of unique human beings. Many genes are subtly different from one individual to another, accounting for much of the variation in our species. These variants are polymorphisms. Polymorphisms are alterations found in DNA in at least 1% of the population. Polymorphisms can be associated with a certain disease, but almost never do they cause the condition.

Mutations are permanent, structural changes in a gene. They may be pathogenic (deleterious, causing disease), of unknown significance, or polymorphic. The redundancy in the genetic code means that not all mutations interfere with protein translation, and not all proteins made from a mutated gene are dysfunctional. Mutations can be somatic, randomly occurring in a cell. These types of mutations cannot be passed onto offspring. Other mutations occur in the germline. Germline mutations are present in every cell in the body, including the oocytes and spermatocytes, and can be passed onto offspring. An inherited germline mutation in a tumor suppressor gene is the most common way that cancer is transmitted within a family.

Genetic Counseling

A genetic counselor is a healthcare professional with training in medical genetics and counseling techniques. This is a rather young field of practice. However, within the past 10 years genetic counseling has been recognized by numerous professional societies as a critical element in the assessment and treatment of patients with or at risk for hereditary cancer syndromes [1–5].

Genetic counseling is a process of identification, education, facilitation, and psychosocial support for the patient and his or her family members. The National Society of Genetic Counselors states that "the purpose of cancer genetic counseling is to educate clients about their chance of developing cancer, help them derive personal meaning form cancer genetic information, and empower them to make educated, informed decisions about genetic testing, cancer screening, and cancer prevention [6]." In addition to educating and empowering patients to make decisions, genetic counselors also assess psychosocial issues that may arise for patients or their families while going through this process.

Referring to a Genetic Counselor

A referral is made to a genetic counselor to determine if a patient and his or her family is at risk for an inherited cancer syndrome and to facilitate suitable genetic testing. The referral is made because something in the patient's presentation, such as family history or disease phenotype, is suggestive of an inherited syndrome. General features of a hereditary cancer syndrome that may prompt a referral to a genetic counselor are listed in Table 2.1.

Family history of cancer is an important risk factor that should be assessed by practitioners caring for patients with cancer. Over a 2-month period in six gastroenterology practices Dudley-Brown and Freivogel found that 26% of patients were at risk of a syndrome of hereditary colorectal cancer, establishing the absolute need for routine family histories [7]. In a less selected group, Mitchell et al. reported that almost 10% of patients had a first-degree relative with colorectal cancer and almost 30% has a first- or second-degree relative affected [8].

In the primary care office, or at the cancer specialist, the family history alone is usually enough to trigger a referral for genetic counseling. Sometimes hereditary cancer features are obscured by lack of knowledge, lack of accuracy, or small family size. Several studies in primary care, surgical, and oncologic practices show that family history of cancer is taken in a low percentage of cases [9–11]. Within a primary care setting one study showed that presence or absence of a family history of cancer was documented in 97.8% of patients' records, but that insufficient information was available to perform a risk assessment in 69.5% of cases [12]. In another report, Mitchell et al. estimated that most patients underestimate their cancer family history, with a sensitivity of 57% for first-degree relatives and 27% for second-degree [13]. However, a family history screening question for colorectal cancer "has anyone in your family ever had cancer or polyps of the colon or rectum" was found to be over 90% accurate in a study of colorectal surgical patients subject to a thorough three-generation pedigree [9]. This question is therefore the bare minimum. Any positive answer should lead to a three-generation family tree with all cancers listed.

Table 2.1 Hallmark feature of hereditary cancer syndromes

Early age at cancer diagnosis (e.g. breast cancer before age 50)
Multiple generation affected with cancer
Multiple primary cancers in an individual
Bilateral or multisynchronous cancers
Clustering of genetically related cancer (e.g. uterine and colon cancer)
Rare cancers (e.g. male with breast cancer)
Known deleterious mutation present in the family

Occasionally, the disease phenotype is suggestive of inheritance. For example, the presence of more than 100 synchronous colorectal adenomas means a polyposis syndrome is present. Oligopolyposis, where patients have less than 100 but more than 10 synchronous adenomas, raises the possibilities of attenuated familial adenomatous polyposis and *MuTYH*-associated polyposis. Genetic counseling and genetic testing for a germline *APC* or *MuTYH* mutation is indicated for all these scenarios.

Personal Medical History

During a counseling session, information is collected on all major illnesses, surgical history, history of benign and malignant tumors, biopsy history, reproductive history, environmental exposures, and cancer surveillance [14]. For patients with a personal history of cancer, information is collected on the site and stage of the cancer, treatment and outcomes, and age at diagnosis. Cancer pathology is also a critical factor. As an example, in hereditary breast ovarian cancer syndrome it has been found that women with a "triple negative" cancer (negative for estrogen-receptor, progesterone-receptor, and HER2) are candidates for *BRCA1* and *BRCA2* testing, even in the absence of a family history of breast or ovarian cancer [15].

Family Medical History

A genetic counselor is trained to obtain a detailed three- to four-generation family history. In taking the history, particular attention is paid to the site and pathology of the cancer, the stage of the cancer, treatment and outcomes, and age at diagnosis. Information is also collected about nonmalignant features of hereditary cancer syndromes. For example, when evaluating a family for Cowden syndrome, in addition to collecting family history of cancer, information is recorded about head circumference and benign dermatologic, thyroid, breast, and endometrial disease. Medical records and/or death certificates are typically requested in order to confirm the diagnoses within the family. For the genetic family history, it is also important to collect information on unaffected family members and deceased family members including age at death and cause of death. Information about ethnicity and consanguinity is also collected on all patients. For patients who have been adopted or have no information about their family medical history, counseling is based on the personal risk factors.

Risk Assessment

Once the personal medical and family history is obtained, a differential diagnosis is established. Various risk assessment models have been established for some of the more common syndromes such as hereditary breast ovarian cancer syndrome [16–21] and hereditary non-polyposis colorectal cancer [22–26]. These models are used to quantify the risk of identifying a mutation in a patient. Upon this assessment, a testing strategy is devised. The patient is counseled on the disease(s) in question in a manner that is tailored to the patient's education level and focused on conveying the necessary information to make an informed decision regarding genetic testing.

In addition to facilitating the patient's understanding of his or her own risks, the genetic counselor helps the patient to identify the family members who may be at risk. A list of the more common hereditary cancer syndromes and their inheritance is listed in Table 2.2. Almost all cancer syndromes follow an autosomal dominant inheritance pattern. This means that an affected individual has a 50% chance of

Table 2.2 Syndromes of hereditary cancer

Syndrome	Genes	Inheritance	Clinical testing available
Ataxia telangiectasia	*ATM*	Recessive (only carriers at risk for cancer)	Yes
Birt-Hogg-Dube syndrome	*BHD*	Dominant	Yes
Carney complex	*PRKRA1*	Dominant	Yes
Familial adenomatous polyposis	*APC*	Dominant	Yes
Familial malignant melanoma	*TP16*	Dominant	Yes
Familial paraganglioma syndrome	*SDHB SDHC SDHD*	Dominant	Yes
Fanconi anemia	*FANCA FANCB FANCC FANCD FANCE FANCF FANCG FANCL*	Recessive	Yes
Gorlin syndrome	*PTCH*	Dominant	Yes
Hereditary breast ovarian cancer	*BRCA1 BRCA2*	Dominant	Yes
Hereditary diffuse gastric cancer	*CDH1*	Dominant	Yes
Hereditary leiomyomatosis and renal cell carcinoma	*FH*	Dominant	Yes
Hereditary papillary renal cell carcinoma	*MET*	Dominant	Yes
Hyperparathyroid-jaw tumor syndrome	*HPRT2*	Dominant	Yes
Juvenile polyposis syndrome	*BMPRIA SMAD4*	Dominant	Yes
Li-Fraumeni syndrome	*P53*	Dominant	Yes
Lynch syndrome	*hMLH1 hMSH2 hMSH6 hPMS2*	Dominant	Yes
Multiple endocrine neoplasia 1	*MEN1*	Dominant	Yes
Multiple endocrine neoplasia 2	*RET*	Dominant	Yes
MuTYH-associated polyposis	*MuTYH*	Recessive	Yes
Neurofibromatosis type 1	*NF1*	Dominant	Yes
Neurofibromatosis type 2	*NF2*	Dominant	Yes
Peutz-Jehgers syndrome	*STK11*	Dominant	Yes
PTEN-hamartoma tumor syndrome	*PTEN*	Dominant	Yes

(continued)

Table 2.2 (continued)

Syndrome	Genes	Inheritance	Clinical testing available
Retinoblastoma	*RB1*	Dominant	Yes
Tuberous sclerosis complex	*TSC1 TSC2*	Dominant	Yes
Von Hippel Lindau disease	*VHL*	Dominant	Yes
Wilms tumor	*WT1*	Dominant	Yes
Xeroderma pigmentosa	*XPA ERCC3 XPC ERCC2 XPE ERCC4 ERCC5*	Recessive	Yes

passing on the pathogenic mutation to each pregnancy. There is also a 50% chance that the mutation would not be passed on.

There are also a few hereditary cancer syndromes that follow an autosomal recessive pattern of inheritance. Autosomal recessive inheritance requires that both copies of the gene are mutated in order for the syndrome to manifest. When both parents are carriers of a mutated gene each offspring has a 25% chance of being unaffected, a 50% chance of also being a carrier, and a 25% chance of inheriting both mutated copies of the gene. In this case, that individual would be affected with the disease.

Genetic Testing

Genetic testing is an important part of the care of families with hereditary cancer syndromes. Ideally, testing is performed on a member of the family who has been diagnosed with cancer. Prior to ordering genetic testing, patients should be fully informed of the risks, benefits, and limitations of genetic testing. As part of this conversation, patients should be aware of the type of testing being ordered, the associated cost, and the turnaround time. Patients should be counseled about the outcomes of testing, and a plan should be established for how results will be disclosed. It is the role of a genetic counselor to ensure that all these issues are properly addressed with the patient.

In 1997, Giardiello et al. showed what can happen when genetic counseling is not a part of genetic testing [27]. They reported on *APC* testing in 177 patients from 125 families during 1995. Only 18.6% (33 of 177) received genetic counseling before the test, and only 16.9% (28 of 166) provided written informed consent. The ordering physicians misinterpreted the test results 31.6% of the time. Finally, when the indications for testing were not those commonly used, the rate of positive results was only 2.3% (1 of 44). While these results are concerning, they apply to a relatively simple monogenic syndrome, with clear dominant inheritance, and penetrance close to 100%. Almost all other syndromes of hereditary cancer are more complex.

Clinical Versus Research Genetic Testing

Important distinctions should be made between clinical and research genetic testing. Clinical genetic testing is used for diagnostic purposes and to guide medical management [28]. Within the United States, clinical testing must be preformed in a laboratory with Clinical Laboratory Improvement Amendments (CLIA) certification. CLIA certification requires that laboratory meets quality control and proficiency testing standards. This certification is a regulation of the Centers for Medical & Medicaid Services, which sets the precedent for other third party payers. There is a charge associated with clinical testing, and the majority of health insurance providers do cover some portion of genetic testing. Additionally, clinical test results are reported in writing. Research testing is done to develop a clinical test or gain a better understanding of a condition [28]. Typically, there is no cost to the patient for research testing as the investigator usually covers this. Research laboratories are neither required to have CLIA certification nor are they obligated to provide patients with the results of research genetic testing. If a patient does receive results from a research study, that information cannot be used to diagnose or manage the patient until it is confirmed in a laboratory with CLIA certification.

Genetic Test Results

For the first family member who undergoes genetic testing, there are three potential results: positive, negative, or uncertain.

A positive result means that a deleterious mutation has been identified thus confirming that the patient has a hereditary cancer syndrome. This result can then be used to direct medical management for that patient and can be used to perform predictive testing for other family members.

A negative result means that no mutation was identified. There are multiple explanations for this result. One explanation is that the patient does not have the genetic syndrome in question. A second explanation is that there are limitations of genetic testing technology. There is always a possibility that a mutation could be present within the gene that could not be detected with current genetic testing technology. Third, there could be a mutation in another gene that is responsible for the cancer in the family. Additionally, if the first person tested in the family is not someone who has been diagnosed with cancer, it is possible that a mutation is present in the family but that individual did not inherit the mutation. It is not possible to distinguish between these possibilities. Therefore, negative genetic test results do not necessarily rule out the possibility that a patient has a hereditary cancer syndrome. In the case of a negative genetic test result, the patient should be counseled that the likelihood that he or she has a hereditary cancer syndrome has been greatly reduced.

Finally, a variant of uncertain significance could be identified. In this case, a genetic alteration has been identified but insufficient data exist in order to determine if this mutation is pathogenic or polymorphic. In general, it is not recommended to perform predictive testing for at-risk family members for variants of uncertain significance.

Predictive Genetic Testing

The results of predictive testing are much more straightforward to interpret. Once a deleterious mutation is identified in a patient, single site testing for that mutation should be offered to all at-risk relatives. Any relative found to have the family-specific deleterious mutation as has the hereditary cancer syndrome in question, that individual should then be offered increased cancer surveillance, chemoprevention, and/or prophylactic surgical options. If a relative is found not to have the family-specific mutation then he or she does not have the hereditary cancer syndrome in question and is at the general population risk to develop cancer. This is considered a "true negative" result. This individual should be offered general population cancer surveillance.

Benefits of Genetic Testing

Identification of a pathogenic mutation provides the patient with an explanation for their personal and/or family history of cancer, allows for medical management options to reduce the risk of developing a future cancer, and makes predictive testing available for family members. If a family member is found to have the family-specific mutation then he or she would be offered increased cancer surveillance and, potentially, prophylactic surgery to help reduce the risk of developing a cancer. Relatives who are affected can be diagnosed early, often before cancer has developed. If a relative is found not to carry the deleterious mutation then he or she would not need to undergo increased surveillance above the general population. This is perhaps the most important advantage of genetic testing, as without it everyone in the family must undergo surveillance as if they were affected. Affected patients can consider their status and the risk to their children in planning a family. Additionally, family planning options such as pre-implantation genetic diagnosis or prenatal testing could be considered if the family-specific mutation has been identified.

Knowledge of the precise location of the mutation and the particular gene involved may allow for prediction of the clinical expression of the disease, and a tailored surveillance program. For example, multiple endocrine neoplasia (MEN) type 2B is the most aggressive form of MEN 2 and is associated with onset of medullary thyroid cancer in the teenage years, pheochromocytoma, and developmental defects. Greater than 95% of patients with MEN 2B have the mutation M918T in exon 15. Current consensus is that patients with this mutation undergo prophylactic thyroidectomy within the first six months of life [29].

Limitations of Genetic Testing

The major limitation of genetic testing is the mutation detection frequency. With the exception of *VHL* gene testing, there is no genetic test for hereditary cancer syndromes that has a 100% mutation detection rate. However, the evolution of genetic testing, with increased sensitivity and mutation detection frequency, has been relatively quick over the last 10 years. While a patient may undergo genetic testing that is negative, or uninformative, it is likely that as sequencing and other genetic testing technologies, such as those to detect large deletions/duplications, are introduced, "mutation negative" patients will have their mutation found. In the case of Peutz-Jeghers syndrome, sequencing of *STK11* will detect 39–69% of mutations. Until 2005, it was believed that a second susceptibility locus existed but then it was found that nearly 30% of patients have large deletions, which would not be detected using sequencing [30]. Now, with the incorporation of large deletion analysis, the deleterious mutation will be identified for the majority of patients with Peutz-Jeghers syndrome.

Risks Associated with Genetic Testing

Some patients and families may wish not to know their hereditary status. This "fear of knowing" is more common in hereditary syndromes without adequate treatment or interventions, such as Li-Fraumeni syndrome. Ideally, through the process of genetic counseling patients will gain an understanding of their cancer risk, strategies to help reduce this risk, and receive psychosocial support for coping with this result.

There is also a possibility that through testing multiple family members nonpaternity could be uncovered. Additionally, patients could learn that they are not biologically related to their family members, as in cases of adoption.

Finally, as long as genetic testing has been offered there has been a fear that the results will be used to influence decisions of employability or insurability. In practice, genetic discrimination is uncommon, and in many syndromes disease phenotype and family history make the diagnosis as clearly as the results of genetic testing. To date, there are no well-documented cases of insurance discrimination with regard to genetic information that have been reported. Further, the Health Insurance Portability and Accountability Act has a provision, which states that genetic testing information cannot be used as a pre-existing condition for patients who are in group health insurance plans. In May 2008, the Genetic Information Nondiscrimination Act (GINA) was signed into law. GINA prohibits United States' insurance companies and employers from discriminating on the basis of genetic information. Genetic information is broadly defined as family history of a disease (up to a fourth-degree relative), genetic services, genetic test results, and participation in research involving genetics. In addition, under this law, insurers and employers are not allowed to request or demand a genetic test. The ability to obtain life and disability insurance are not protected by any laws.

Conclusion

Diagnosing a hereditary cancer syndrome is essential for management of patients and their family members. To achieve the best outcome for patients, identification, assessment, diagnosis, and management requires a multidisciplinary team. A key member of the team is the genetic counselor. Genetic counselors are healthcare providers trained to obtain and evaluate medical and family histories; explain the genetics of hereditary cancer syndromes; facilitate genetic testing; interpret and discuss the results of genetic testing, and advise about genetic discrimination and family planning.

References

1. Recommendations from the EGAPP Working Group: genetic testing strategies in newly diagnosed individuals with colorectal cancer aimed at reducing morbidity and mortality from Lynch syndrome in relatives. *Genet Med* **11**, 35–41 (2009).
2. Khatcheressian, J.L. et al. American Society of Clinical Oncology 2006 update of the breast cancer follow-up and management guidelines in the adjuvant setting. *J Clin Oncol* **24**, 5091–7 (2006).
3. Lancaster, J.M. et al. Society of Gynecologic Oncologists Education Committee statement on risk assessment for inherited gynecologic cancer predispositions. *Gynecol Oncol* **107**, 159–62 (2007).
4. Murphy, C.D. et al. The American Cancer Society guidelines for breast screening with magnetic resonance imaging: an argument for genetic testing. *Cancer* **113**, 3116–20 (2008).
5. Winawer, S. et al. Colorectal cancer screening and surveillance: clinical guidelines and rationale-Update based on new evidence. *Gastroenterology* **124**, 544–60 (2003).
6. Trepanier, A. et al. Genetic cancer risk assessment and counseling: recommendations of the national society of genetic counselors. *J Genet Couns* **13**, 83–114 (2004).
7. Dudley-Brown, S. & Freivogel, M. Hereditary colorectal cancer in the gastroenterology clinic: how common are at-risk patients and how do we find them? *Gastroenterol Nurs* **32**, 8–16 (2009).
8. Mitchell, R.J. et al. Accuracy of reporting of family history of colorectal cancer. *Gut* **53**, 291–5 (2004).
9. Church, J. & McGannon, E. Family history of colorectal cancer: how often and how accurately is it recorded? *Dis Colon Rectum* **43**, 1540–4 (2000).
10. Lynch, H.T. et al. Who should be sent for genetic testing in hereditary colorectal cancer syndromes? *J Clin Oncol* **25**, 3534–42 (2007).
11. Murff, H.J., Spigel, D.R. & Syngal, S. Does this patient have a family history of cancer? An evidence-based analysis of the accuracy of family cancer history. *JAMA* **292**, 1480–9 (2004).
12. Tyler, C.V., Jr. & Snyder, C.W. Cancer risk assessment: examining the family physician's role. *J Am Board Fam Med* **19**, 468–77 (2006).
13. Mitchell, R.J. et al. Prevalence of family history of colorectal cancer in the general population. *Br J Surg* **92**, 1161–4 (2005).
14. Schneider, K.A. *Counseling About Cancer: Strategies for Genetic Counseling*, 333 (Wiley-Liss, Inc., New York, 2002).
15. Young, S.R. et al. The prevalence of BRCA mutations among young women with triple-negative breast cancer. *BMC Cancer* **9**, 86 (2009).
16. Berry, D.A., Parmigiani, G., Sanchez, J., Schildkraut, J. & Winer, E. Probability of carrying a mutation of breast-ovarian cancer gene BRCA1 based on family history. *J Natl Cancer Inst* **89**, 227–38 (1997).

17. Couch, F.J. et al. BRCA1 mutations in women attending clinics that evaluate the risk of breast cancer. *N Engl J Med* **336**, 1409–15 (1997).
18. Frank, T.S. et al. Clinical characteristics of individuals with germline mutations in BRCA1 and BRCA2: analysis of 10,000 individuals. *J Clin Oncol* **20**, 1480–90 (2002).
19. Shattuck-Eidens, D. et al. BRCA1 sequence analysis in women at high risk for susceptibility mutations. Risk factor analysis and implications for genetic testing. *JAMA* **278**, 1242–50 (1997).
20. Stoppa-Lyonnet, D. et al. BRCA1 sequence variations in 160 individuals referred to a breast/ovarian family cancer clinic. Institut Curie Breast Cancer Group. *Am J Hum Genet* **60**, 1021–30 (1997).
21. Tyrer, J., Duffy, S.W. & Cuzick, J. A breast cancer prediction model incorporating familial and personal risk factors. *Stat Med* **23**, 1111–30 (2004).
22. Balmana, J. et al. Prediction of MLH1 and MSH2 mutations in Lynch syndrome. *JAMA* **296**, 1469–78 (2006).
23. Barnetson, R.A. et al. Identification and survival of carriers of mutations in DNA mismatch-repair genes in colon cancer. *N Engl J Med* **354**, 2751–63 (2006).
24. Chen, S. et al. Prediction of germline mutations and cancer risk in the Lynch syndrome. *JAMA* **296**, 1479–87 (2006).
25. Marroni, F. et al. A genetic model for determining MSH2 and MLH1 carrier probabilities based on family history and tumor microsatellite instability. *Clin Genet* **69**, 254–62 (2006).
26. Wijnen, J.T. et al. Clinical findings with implications for genetic testing in families with clustering of colorectal cancer. *N Engl J Med* **339**, 511–8 (1998).
27. Giardiello, F.M. et al. The use and interpretation of commercial APC gene testing for familial adenomatous polyposis. *N Engl J Med* **336**, 823–7 (1997).
28. GeneTests. Medical Genetics Information Resource. (University of Seattle, Washington, 1993–2009).
29. Brandi, M.L. et al. Guidelines for diagnosis and therapy of MEN type 1 and type 2. *J Clin Endocrinol Metab* **86**, 5658–71 (2001).
30. Aretz, S. et al. High proportion of large genomic STK11 deletions in Peutz-Jeghers syndrome. *Hum Mutat* **26**, 513–9 (2005).

Chapter 3
An *Ethos* of Genetic Testing

Roy E. Gandy and Charles B. Rodning

It was the best of times, it was the worst of times, it was the age of wisdom, it was the age of foolishness, it was the epoch of belief, it was the epoch of incredulity, it was the season of light, it was the season of darkness, it was the spring of hope, it was the winter of despair, we had everything before us, we had nothing before us, we were all going direct to Heaven, we were all going direct the other way-in short, the period was so far like the present period, that some of its noisiest authorities insisted on its being received, for good or for evil, in the superlative degree of comparison only.
Chapter I, Book I, *A Tale of Two Cities* Charles Dickens (1812–1870) [1].

Overview

1. The biotechnological revolution in genetics and genetic testing poses ethical dilemmas for patients, families, health care providers, scientists, humanists (sacred and secular), employers, insurers, and governmental agencies.
2. We propose an aretological (virtue-based) ethical principlism (intentionalistic) and the Four-Way Test (consequentialistic) as rational, philosophical, and jurisprudential models to deliberate and balance conflicting constituencies and contingencies.

   Note that issues related to each stratification *vide infra* are cumulative.

3. Genetic Testing: Adults

   - individual versus family
   - autonomy versus responsibility

4. Genetic Testing: Children

   - parent versus child
   - autonomy versus privacy/confidentiality
   - vulnerability

R.E. Gandy (✉)
Department of Surgery, University of South Alabama Medical Center, Mobile, AL 36617, USA
e-mail: rgandy@usouthal.edu

C.N. Ellis (ed.), *Inherited Cancer Syndromes: Current Clinical Management*,
DOI 10.1007/978-1-4419-6821-0_3, © Springer Science+Business Media, LLC 2011

5. Genetic Testing: Fetus (Pre-Natal)

   - ensoulment/personhood
   - pregnancy termination

6. Genetic Testing: Embryo (Pre-Implantation)

   - selection or deselection for gender, endowments (physical, mental), or immu-
     nological compatibility with other offspring – using an embryo/child as a
     means to an end

7. Genetic Testing: Commercialization, direct-to-consumer marketing, scientific
   validity, and interpretability regulation.
8. The indicative plus the imperative equals the normative.

Reflective citizens of every society have probably perceived that they have existed
on the cusp of an ethical and a moral twilight from the ravages of the Four
Horsemen of the Apocalypse. Futurists argue that *Homo sapiens sapiens* has
recently entered the age of biotechnology, having experienced the hunter–gatherer
age (eons of time in duration), the agrarian age (millennia), the industrial age
(centuries), and the information age (decades). The era of biotechnology is marked
by numerous scientific and humanistic endeavors including the human genome
project; genetic engineering, cloning, and longevity; stem cell research; expansion
of the *materia medica* and instrumentality; xenotransplantation; and the intersec-
tion of medical economics, politics, and medicolegal issues at the local, national,
and international levels [2]. Those endeavors could be characterized as Herculean
feats, of Promethean proportions, but with Faustain bargainable implications.

A relevant and germane semantic distinction exists between the terms ethics and
morals: ethics (Gk., *ethika*, L., *ethica*) denotes "character;" and morals (L., *moralis*)
denotes "usage," "mood," "custom," or "behavior". Fundamentally, ethics is intra-
mental, potential, and intentional, whereas morals are extramental, actualized, and
consequential. Normative – evaluatory and clarificatory – ethics connotes a methodology for analyzing the standards and criteria of rules and judgments regarding
right and wrong/good and bad character and behavior [3, 4].

Health Care Ethics: Groundwork

R. D. Orr has referred to the discipline of health care ethics as deliberative, nuanced, and
subtle reflections upon ambiguity and uncertainty [5]. He and the present authors
perceive that such reflection must be rationally, philosophically, and jurisprudentially
grounded. The authors advocate application of an aretological (Gk., "virtue-based") ethical
principlist methodology to the analysis of inherited cancer syndromes [3, 4]. Theoretically
and pragmatically, the doctrine of virtue-based (L., *virtus*, "excellence," "manly," "mas-
terly") principlism incorporates the cardinal (courage, justice, prudence, and temperance)
and the theological (faith, hope, and charity) virtues as predicated upon the:

- natural law (L., *lex naturalis*) of Socrates, Plato [6], Aristotle [7], Zeno, Epictetus [8], Marcus Tullis Cicero [9], Lucius Annaeus Seneca [10], and Marcus Aurelius Antonis Augustus [11];
- law of reason (L., *lex ratio*) of Saint Augustine of Hippo [12] and Saint Thomas Aquinas [13]; and
- moral law within (L., *lex intus moralis*) of Epicuris, Titus Lucretius Carus [14], John Locke [15], and Immanuel Kant [16–18].

Pragmatically and productively, aretological ethical principlism overarches and complements the concordant and correspondent ethical systems of deontology (Gk., *deon*, "obligations," "duty" – a process, intention) as predicated upon the philosophies of the Torah and Thomas Hobbes [19]; teleology (Gk., *telos*, "purpose," "end" – a result, consequence) as predicated upon the philosophies of the Holy Gospel and Niccolo Machiavelli [20]; utilitarianism (L., *utilitas*, "useful") as predicated upon the philosophies of Jeremy Bentham [21] and John Stuart Mill [22]; and axiology (Gk., *axia*, "value" "worth") as predicated upon the philosophers cited *vide supra* and the philosophies of Max Weber [23] and John Dewey [24]. The authors acknowledge that their advocacy of aretological ethical principlism is Occidental, subjective, qualitative, experiential, *a posteriori*, derivative, and logically contingent (conditional), rather than objective, quantitative, experimental, *a priori, sui generis*, and logically necessary. Nevertheless, the authors argue *a fortiori* that aretological ethical principlism provides an apprehensible and a rational, philosophical, and jurisprudential grounding for analyses and deliberations of potential ethical dilemmas. The authors would also argue that since aretological ethical principlism is grounded upon a syncretic (eclectic and synthetic) philosophical Ciceronian system [9], that it is both universalizable and particular and provides a coherence, correspondence, concordance, clarity, concision, and commensurability to ethical deliberations and analyses.

Aretological ethical principlism segues with the expostulations of Sir W. D. Ross in his monograph *The Right and the Good* [25]. He argued that individuals interact with their community in the context of the following *prima facie* (L., "at first sight," "self-evident") intra- and inter-personal duties:

- autonomy: *voluntas aegroti suprema lex* (L., "right of choice...");
- beneficence: *salus aegroti suprema lex* (L., "help others...");
- nonmaleficence: *primum non nocere* (L., "first do no harm");
- justice: *justitia* (L., "just," "fair") balance of personal happiness and duty;
- honesty/integrity: truthfulness of disclosure;
- fidelity: fulfillment of promises/agreements;
- reparation: compensation for wrongful acts;
- gratitude: recompense;
- dignity: *dignitatis humane* (L., "human worthiness");
- self-improvement: help oneself;
- liberty: non-coercion; and
- responsibility: contribution to the commonwealth.

A balance between self-assertive and integrative behavior was emphasized, in the context of the numerous social relationships by which humankind defines itself existentially.

Ethical analyses of experimental and clinical health care are also informed by jurisprudential and professional guidelines, which have emerged since the mid-Twentieth Century in response to historical barbarity. The Nuremberg Code (Nuremberg Military Tribunal…, 1947) [26], the Declaration of Helsinki (World Medical Association, 1964) [27], the Belmont Report (National Commission for the Protection of Human Subjects of Biomedical and Behavioral Research, 1979) [28], and the International Ethical Guidelines for Biomedical Research Involving Human Subjects (Council for International Organizations of Medical Sciences and the World Health Organization, 1982, 1993) [29], are considered primary sources, which adjudicated specific historical events. As articulated by R. J. Levine [30] and E. J. Emanuel et al. [31], seven requirements for translational clinical research and, by extension, for humanistic clinical care, emerged from those deliberations, which systematically elucidated the fundamental protections cumulatively embedded in the basic philosophy of those documents:

• social and scientific value;
• scientific validity;
• equitable subject selection;
• favorable risk-to-benefit ratio;
• independent review;
• informed consent; and
• respect for enrollees.

The intent of the aforementioned is to balance the dualities and dichotomies of is and ought, free will and determinism, self and society, individual and community, freedom and responsibility, parent and child, patient and family, patient and health care providers, subject and researcher, science and humanities, experimental and clinical, the sacred and the profane, and life and death. Since all rational human endeavor involves risk-benefit, cost-benefit, and effort-yield analyses, the Law of Parsimony (William of Ockham) [32] and the Law of Unintended Consequences (Aristotle) [7] must be acknowledged. Accordingly, the authors advocate *sensus commonalis* when applying these tenets to health care ethical deliberations of genetic testing for inherited cancer syndromes.

Operationally and productively, aretological ethical principlism (intentionalistic) and the Four-Way Test [33] (consequentialistic) provides a means to achieve balance, proportionality, and moderation – *auris mediocratus* (L., "the golden mean") – within ethical deliberations:

• Is it true?
• Is it fair?
• Will it generate goodwill?
• Will it be beneficial?

The apothegm – the indicative plus the imperative equals the normative – applies.

Genetic Testing: Adults

A genetic basis for an increasing number of inherited cancer syndromes has been discovered in recent years. Genetic tests have become readily available for several somatic and germline mutations, permitting risk assessment of asymptomatic patients in cancer prone families. This information has substantial potential to improve clinical management, but also poses substantial health care ethical dilemmas within legal, social, and economic frameworks. Deliberation of those issues intersects among patients, families, communities, health care providers, researchers, and public health advocates.

As mentioned, normative ethics encompasses a systematic examination of the moral aspects of the human condition. Ideally, health care ethics should systematically analyze ethical issues in the domains of clinical care and research. The major foci of health care ethics include experimentation, equitable distribution of resources, patient-health care provider relationships, public health and welfare, and preventive medicine. Robust ongoing discussions and debates related to genetic testing in inherited cancer syndromes intersect with each of those domains as reflected by a voluminous academic and popular literature.

In 1983 the *President's Commission for the Study of Ethical Problems in Medical and Biomedical Behavioral Research* reported its recommendations regarding genetic screening [34]. That report emphasized the imperatives of autonomy, confidentiality, informed consent, and non-discrimination, which have been pivotal to health care ethical deliberations in the interim. Emerging and available technology for genetic screening has heightened awareness that the results of those tests may substantially impact upon individual patients, their families, and their communities, since results may affect health care decisions for both individuals and others. The Presidential Commission Report [34] advised that medical genetics programs should promulgate specific procedural guidelines that incorporate rational, philosophical, ethical, and legal principles regarding the performance and application of those tests:

- individual patient information and results should not be disseminated without explicit informed consent; and
- genetic tissue and data archival storage repositories should ensure anonymity of donors.

Those recommendations address one dichotomy – that although the results of genetic testing may guide surveillant, diagnostic, and therapeutic decisions, including reproductive, those findings could potentially result in discrimination by communities, employers, insurance carriers, and governmental agencies.

Those recommendations are predicated upon the concepts of patient autonomy and confidentiality, which are steeped in Occidental tradition (Oath of Hippocrates [35]). Contemporary common, civil, statutory, and constitutional law acknowledges those precedents, and health care providers may be culpable and liable for unauthorized disclosure. A counterpoint, however, is a need to balance fiduciary duties to a patient and a need to prevent harm to others. For example, what if a patient requested that their relatives not be informed of the results of genetic testing, despite the fact that those relatives could be afflicted? The Presidential Commission Report [34] advised that violation of patient autonomy and confidentiality would be justified to prevent harm to others, a recommendation supported by The Institute of Medicine (1994); The American Society of Human Genetics (1998); and the Ethical, Legal, and Social Implications (ELSI) Program/National Center for Human Genome Research (2001) [36]. The imperatives in that regard include:

- failed efforts to persuade a patient to share information voluntarily;
- high probability of harm to uninformed relatives;
- confidence that the information, if known, could avoid harm;
- harm would be grievous; and
- only relevant genetic information should be disclosed.

The Presidential Commission Report [34] also concluded that informed consent for genetic screening should be conditional upon approval to disclose information that might indicate cancer risks for relatives. It concluded that confidentiality was not an absolute right, and that health care providers and the State have a duty to protect others from harm (L., *primum non nocere*).

There is also the issue of anonymity related to the archival storage of tissue and data from genetic analyses. The requirement that storage repositories retain large amounts of genetic material and data would certainly be useful in ongoing genetic research for many medical conditions. If information from those repositories were disseminated, would it violate a patient's and family's privacy and otherwise harm them in terms of social opportunities, employability, and insurability? What if information from future testing indicated potential harm? Should patients and families be notified of newly discovered risks?

The "duty to disclose" to patients has been recognized judicially. Several adjudications have concluded that physicians have a duty to breach confidentiality and warn those exposed to harm. *In re* Safer v. Pack involved litigation by a patient's daughter 25 years after treatment of her father's colon cancer. When she developed colon cancer, she obtained slides of her father's specimens, which revealed familial adenomatous/polypasis coli (FAP) and cancer. A suit was filed against the surgeon's estate for breach of "duty to disclose," more specifically, failing to warn the daughter that she may develop cancer. The court ruled in favor of the plaintiff [Safer v. Pack, 677 A. 2d 1188 (N.J. App), appeal denied 683 A. zd 1163 (N.J. 1966)]. *In re* Pate v. Threlkel concerned a child's suit against a physician who treated her mother's medullary thyroid cancer. It alleged negligence for not warning the child about possibly developing cancer. The court ruled that a "duty to disclose" was incumbent upon a physician. Nevertheless, the court concluded that the duty had been fulfilled by warning the patient's mother and thereby ruled in favor of the defense [Pate v. Threlkel 661 So. 2d 278 (Fla. 1995)]. *In re* Tarasoff v. Regents imposed a duty upon therapists to warn potential victims that a mentally disturbed patient had verbalized that he "might kill someone." The ruling implied a duty to break the confidentiality of the therapeutic relationship and a "duty to disclose" to persons at risk for harm external to that relationship. The court ruled in favor of the plaintiff [Tarasoff v. Regents of the University of California 17 CAL 3rd 425; 551 p. 2 of 334 (1976)].

Additionally, the Presidential Commission Report [34] advised states to modify their respective adoption laws, to ensure that information about genetic risks could be conveyed to adoptees or their biologic families if serious harm was possible, i.e. limited unsealing of adoption data. The aforementioned emphasizes that health care ethical deliberations are informed by cognizance of guidelines issued by professional organizations and by legal precedents.

A typical clinical encounter may serve to illustrate the imperative of informed consent. A patient consults her physician when she learns her brother has undergone an operation for colon cancer and colonic polyps. Specifically, she seeks advice about genetic testing for herself and her children to determine if an inherited cancer syndrome is present within her family and what should be done if tests detect an inherited cancer associated gene. Genetic counseling would ensure her informed consent (principle of autonomy) based on discussion of anticipated procedures, techniques, indications, risks, benefits, burdens, and alternatives. The principle of autonomy implies a patient's "right" to decide and consent to or refuse the proposed intervention. Informed consent has important ethical and legal dimensions. Allegations may result if patients are dissatisfied with an outcome and seek redress, claiming that inadequate information was provided. Most authorities argue that a patient's decision must be based upon an understanding, utility, and usability of information. Substituted judgments for others, particularly children, also deserve careful analysis and attention regarding genetic tests. For instance, what if a child learns he carries a gene predisposing him to cancer; will that psychological "burden" cause him to resent any "consent" made by parents? Legal concerns and lack of scientific sophistication among the general public may render informed consent documents labor intensive, lengthy, cumbersome, and time-consuming, but essential.

Genetic Testing: Children

As alluded to *vide supra*, genetic testing of children poses additional ethical conundrums. For example, early-onset preventive strategies for FAP such as endoscopic surveillance or proctocolectomy are advisable, since cancer may be clinically expressed before adulthood. Genetic testing of a child in such a family is logical and rational, because interventions exist which would potentially benefit the child if the tests were positive and allay anxiety if the tests were negative. Actual realizable benefit to a child tested remains the most ethically compelling rationale in those circumstances. Decisions for genetic testing of children generally follow a benefit-burden analysis model [37].

What if, however, parents requested genetic testing of their child for adult onset conditions? Many genetic counselors advocate deferring until a child becomes an adult (15–18 years of age). Some parents counter that a child "needs to know" if there are potential health risks, so that strategies can be formulated which could affect career, educational, employment, and marital choices. Health care providers should always clarify the psychological and sociological benefits and burdens that genetic testing may potentially impose. One sequela of the aforementioned scenario would be stigmatization of a child within a family unit, e.g., the "vulnerable child syndrome," whereby parents are overly protective of the afflicted child. Other children within the family may resent increased attention to the positively-tested sibling. Even issues of "who decides?" within a family unit are problematic. Parental authority (autonomy) for health care decisions involving their children has long been culturally and legally normative.

Generally, parents have strong interests in promoting their children's health and welfare and are generally best informed to render health care decisions. The concept of autonomy recognizes the rights of individuals to exercise health care choices *laissez faire*. However, precedent and prudent limits to parental decision-making authority include issues of required immunizations, transfusions, and extraordinary life support measures. Health care providers serve a fiduciary role to protect minors if they perceive parental decisions are not in a child's best interests or are abusive. Conflict resolution in some circumstances consists of simple refusal to conduct a genetic test, consultation with a health care ethics committee, or referral to a domestic civil court to petition for appointment of a *guardian ad litem* for health care decisions [38].

Several states require mandatory newborn genetic screening, recognizing that early diagnosis coupled with timely effective treatment can avoid harms inherent with conditions such as: biotinidase deficiency, congenital hypothyroidism, cystic fibrosis, galactosemia, homocystinuria, maple syrup urine disease, phenylketonuria, and hemoglobinopathies. The Presidential Commission Report [34] advised voluntary genetic screening tests in most circumstances. Mandatory genetic screening was considered ethically justifiable only in situations when clear harm could be avoided and efforts at voluntary screening had failed. That conclusion illustrated a classical ethical dilemma, namely, how to decide between conflicting *prima facie* duties of autonomy (permits parents to voluntarily choose testing) and beneficence (promoting community-wide health benefits and preventing harms). Legally and morally the prevention of harm to vulnerable children has prevailed over parental rights to refuse certain health care recommendations.

Counseling is prudent prior to genetic testing of children. With bilateral dialogue, decisions which are ethically valid can emerge such that "benefits" outweigh "burdens." Many elements are needed for sound decisions. Health care providers must be keenly aware of the science applicable to a particular test and condition; the family pedigree; the goals and dynamics of the child-family unit; and the ability of the latter to comprehend complicated information. They must be cognizant of national guidelines, both ethical and scientific, and relevant legal precedent to ensure that the interests of all are properly proportioned.

Genetic Testing: Fetus (Pre-Natal)

The technical aspects of prenatal genetic testing have become ever more sophisticated. Newer methodologies, such as FISH (fluorescent *in situ* hybridization) or isolation of fetal genetic material from maternal blood, may emerge as less invasive and risky options for prenatal diagnosis of genetic conditions [36]. Those and other methodologies may replace amniocentesis or villus biopsy for prenatal screening methodologies. Prenatal tests that reveal genetic conditions which may represent substantial burdens to the neonate and family, will impose an ethical dilemma for parents. Pregnancy termination *vis-á-vis* burdens of care of the afflicted newborn would need to be discussed, including assessment of family values in the context of aretological ethical principles and legal precedents. Prenatal diagnosis would permit preparation for treatment of a child born with disability and preparation for a safer parturition. Diagnosis of lethal conditions such as anencephaly would permit obstetrical planning for a mother's safety.

By contrast, testing for adult-onset disorders is usually not recommended to families opposed to pregnancy termination, because the information could cause years of stigmatization. Refusal to provide a prenatal test has been a recent topic of ethical debate. The situation discussed involved a couple who had requested genetic testing during their first pregnancy, due to the husband's carrier status for Huntington's chorea (an inherited and fatal neurologic disorder typically expressed during the fourth decade of life). Several respected professional organizations have published guidelines suggesting provision of tests only to patients who have reached adulthood, since there is no effective treatment for that disorder [39].

Another guideline, arguing from another perspective, advises against prenatal testing if a couple plans to complete the pregnancy even if the result is positive. They argue that a decision of an individual upon reaching adulthood supersedes that of a parent [40]. By permitting parents to decide, a child's autonomy and confidentiality (the parents know without his/her permission) have been violated. Alternatively, the Human Genetics Society of Australia, advised that prenatal diagnosis should be available for a high-risk fetus with a genetically identifiable "condition" and that the parents can then decide their course of action with the advice of genetic counselors [41]. Which has the greater priority when these issues are in conflict – a parent's right to know or an offspring's right to decide at maturity?

Other authorities have argued in favor of a more liberal stance regarding prenatal genetic testing. Theoretically it could abrogate anxiety about raising a child in uncertainty and facilitate decisions about future procreation. Some couples would consider any stance against genetic testing as being paternalistic by subordinating their concerns. Might some couples deceive in order to secure tests that they think they are justified in requesting?

The aforementioned examples reflect a central struggle in contemporary health care ethics in relation to prenatal genetic testing – how to balance conflicting duties and principles in a society and health care system which has rendered the option of pregnancy termination legally permissible. Establishment of the time of ensoulment/

personhood during the continuum of zygote, embryo, fetus, neonate, infant, child is unresolved – conception? implantation? parturition? maturation? A child born already labeled with a lethal diagnosis may confront a life of potential discrimination and stigmatization in social and family relationships. Health care ethical guidelines for prenatal testing will evolve *pari passu* with technology. Issues, technical and humanistic, have become so complex that qualified genetic counselors will assume an increasingly important role in such deliberations. Evaluation and clarification of psychosocial and economic issues, uncertainties of test results, and preventive and therapeutic options post-testing, will be pivotal to ensuring responsible and professional use of those tests.

Another issue is what will be the impact of public demand for genetic testing? The principle of justice argues for reasonable and fair allocation of resources by society for genetic testing. Genetic testing services should be provided by modern health care systems and should protect vulnerable patients. More difficult to answer is the level of scientific and public consensus required to establish funded public health programs for genetic testing, particularly among the under- and un-insured. Research is needed to establish the validity and predictability of tests, such that resources are allocated commensurate with available and effective treatment regimens, to prevent harm conferred by inherited cancer syndromes.

Genetic Testing: Embryo (Pre-Implantation)

Pre-implantation genetic diagnosis (PGD) has recently emerged as a technique for detection of inherited cancer syndromes and other abnormalities [42]. *In-vitro* fertilization (IVF) technology is employed. One cell from a blastomere is isolated and analyzed – if positive the embryo is discarded and if negative the embryo is implanted. As alluded to *vide supra* there is no uniform agreement regarding the moral or legal status or standing of an embryo. Non-implantation of an afflicted embryo would not legally constitute pregnancy termination. The aforementioned technology is expensive ($25,000.00) and only partially successful (60%), but an option for couples opposed to pregnancy termination and strongly committed to conception of a child who is without an adverse hereditary health condition. PGD has been recognized by the American Society of Reproductive Medicine as an ethically acceptable option to prevent an inherited cancer syndrome [43].

Since IVF was first introduced in 1978, the number of reproductive clinics performing such services has expanded. A recent review reported that over 7,000 PGD procedures have been performed, which have resulted in over 1,000 live births [44]. Recently PGD testing was approved by the United Kingdom Authority for Human Fertilization and Embryology (HFEA, the licensing agency) for inherited breast and colon cancer syndromes among high-risk patients of the National Health Service. Previously, it had only authorized genetic testing for early onset conditions such as cystic fibrosis [45]. In the United States of America the use of PGD is not covered by private health insurance or publicly funded public health agencies.

More families appear willing to expend discretionary funds for PGD to prevent suffering from inherited cancer syndromes. The goal of preventing harm has ethical propriety. Some authorities worry that expanded indications for PGD might eventually lead to testing for gender selection or "enhancements," such as athleticism or intellectual prowess [46]. Those are legitimate ethical concerns. Advocacy of aretological ethical principlism and the *prima facie* duties of autonomy, beneficence, nonmalfeasance, and justice, would support public funding of PGD in cancer related syndromes, but not for gender selection or enhancement ("designer babies").

Might even fertile couples in the future request PGD as a means to ensure that a cancer gene is not transmitted? Presently, PGD has been used for detection of an increasing number of genes for cancer susceptibility syndromes [46]:

Multiple endocrine neoplasia Type 2 (RET)	Medullary thyroid cancer
Fanconi Anemia (FA)	Leukemia
FANCD l/BRCA 1,2	Breast cancer
MUTYH (autosomal/recessive)	FAP/colon cancer
APC (autosomal/dominant)	FAP/colon cancer
MSH2, MSH6	Colon cancer (HNPCC)
Li-Fraumeni Syndrome (LFS)	Adrenal, brain, and breast cancer
Retinoblastoma	Ocular cancer

PGD has also been used to "select" matched potential siblings for patients with FA or other conditions requiring stem cell transplantation for survival [47]. Should parents "conceive a child to save a child?" Should an embryo be "a lifeboat for the living?" Ethical controversy surrounds that issue from several perspectives. Obviously, the embryo does not consent. A parent's decision is not for the "best interests" of the embryo, but for the family unit and siblings who are "in harm's way." An embryo/child is being used as a means rather than as an end. Regardless of those valid ethical objections, will families continue to pursue that option when confronted with fatal conditions among their living children?

As described, PGD has moved medicine beyond preventing certain genetic diseases, just as immunizations and antibiotic medications reduced morbidity and mortality from infectious diseases. However, at least theoretically, if certain genes can be "selected out" by testing, others can be "selected in," which raises additional ethical concerns. Could this become a "slippery slope" from prevention of harms to gender and trait selection, eugenics, and social engineering [48–50]? In that context health care providers serve as guardians and gatekeepers. Couples requesting PGD will defend their rationale, such as infertility or family history of serious inherited disease, and putatively that information will be analyzed clinically, ethically, and legally before any procedure is authorized. We agree strongly with prevention of harm, and while respecting autonomy in reproductive decisions, we are mindful that society has traditionally constrained such choices. The boundary between autonomy and beneficence is an ongoing debate. In practical terms PGD is expensive and generally not covered by insurance. "Medical tourism" – patients traveling to foreign locations for specific procedures, including PGD – is a new cultural phenomenon.

PGD has also become increasingly recognized as an option for cancer patients who have reduced fertility due to oncologic operations or chemo-irradiation therapies [43]. Who should give informed consent before harvest and cryopreservation of oocytes? – patient?, child?, parent?, spouse? Ovarian tissue preservation, if perfected, may permit restoration of fertility among those who survive cancer syndromes. Nevertheless, that technology is currently considered experimental, and rigorous adherence to guidelines and protocols – scientific and humanistic – is imperative [30, 31].

Genetic Testing: Commercialization

The print and electronic media convey a plethora of information regarding genetics and genetic testing [51]. Direct-to-consumer marketing of genetic testing services and "in the privacy of your own home" genetic tests are an actuality. At present these services and tests are under-regulated by professional or governmental agencies. Results reported are rarely categoric and usually require sophisticated interpretation. Critical analyses of the implications of those services and tests from scientific and humanistic perspectives are essential.

Summary

The Human Genome Project and advances in genetic testing have heightened public awareness about inherited cancer syndromes and attendant health care ethical issues. Although less than 10% of malignant disease is currently thought to be inheritable, emerging genetic testing represents potential opportunities for identifying patients and relatives with such predisposition. Opportunities for genetic screening, prevention, intervention, and surveillance may potentially reduce the incidence/prevalence and lessen morbidity and mortality from those malignant diseases [52].

The authors have argued in favor of an aretological ethical principlism (intentionalistic) and the Four-Way Test (consequentialistic) as foundational health care ethical deliberative methodologies. The *prima facie* duties of autonomy, beneficence, non-malfeasance, justice, honesty/integrity, fidelity, reparation, gratitude, dignity, self-improvement, liberty, and responsibility, provide a valuable conceptual framework for such deliberations. Patients, families, and communities will be substantially affected by ethical dimensions of genetic testing. Health care providers will confront difficult decisions in dealing with families who have a history suggestive of an inheritable cancer syndrome. Health insurance carriers must address appropriate and fair levels of financial coverage for persons who may have an inheritable cancer disorder. State and federal governments and public health agencies must address who will be entitled to genetic testing and whether genetic predispositions to diseases will constitute disability within a legal framework. Researchers will need to address ethical issues related to disclosure of information and the use of archival genetic tissue and data for ongoing research. Reproductive clinics have already seen an increase in the use of IVF and PDG for testing and/or de-selection of embryos likely to express an inheritable cancer syndrome or other inheritable disorder. Pharmaceutical companies are marketing "over-the-counter" genetic tests directly to consumers. Religious organizations are monitoring the aforementioned, often with considerable consternation.

If ethics encompasses a systematic examination of the moral aspects of the human condition, health care ethics systematically studies ethical dilemmas in clinical practice and research, including the domains of experimentation, equitable distribution of resources, patient–health care provider relationships, public health and welfare, and preventive medicine. Within each of those domains there are vigorous and ongoing discussions related to genetic testing in inherited cancer and other syndromes.

Contemporaneously, health care providers have been accused of losing the "old fashioned values of bedside clinical care," tailored to an individual patient's needs and respectful of their values and family contexts. The biotechnological revolution of genetics and genetic testing, will *de facto* mandate that health care providers become even more aware of a patient's values as well as their clinical condition. "Genetics will revolutionize [health care]. It will send it back to its roots; back to its future [52]."

> Cease, then, nor order imperfection name;
> Our proper bliss depends on what we blame.
> Know thy own point: this kind, this due degree
> Of blindness, weakness, Heav'n bestows on thee.
> Submit: in this or any other sphere,
> Secure to be as bless'd as thou canst bear;
> Safe in the hand of one disposing pow'r,
> Or in the natal or the mortal hour.
> All nature is but art, unknown to thee;
> All chance, direction, which thou canst not see;
> All discord, harmony not understood;
> All partial evil, universal good.
> And, spite of pride, in erring reason's spite,
> One truth is clear, '*Whatever is, is right.*'
> Epistle I
> Essay on Man [53]
> Alexander Pope (1688–1744)

Acknowledgements The authors gratefully acknowledge and commend the chapter written by T. F. Ackerman entitled "Ethical Issues in Genetic Testing for Cancer Susceptibility" in the First Edition of this monograph. We also express appreciation to Ms. Betty J. Young-Pledger, Secretary

V, and Ms. Patricia A. Dickinson, Word Processing Specialist, Department of Surgery, College of Medicine and Medical Center University of South Alabama, Mobile, Alabama, for superbly typing our manuscript.

References

1. Dickens CJH. A tale of two cities (1859). New York: Everyman's Library, P. Dutton, Publishers, 1948.
2. Starr P. The social transformation of American medicine. New York: Basic Books, Inc., 1982.
3. Pellegrino ED. Humanism and the physician. Knoxville, Tennessee: University of Tennessee Press, 1979.
4. Pellegrino ED, Thomasma DC. The virtues in medical practice. New York: Oxford University Press, 1993.
5. Orr RD, Chay A. Medical ethics. A primer for students. Bristol, Tennessee: Paul Tournier Institute, Christian Medical and Dental Association, 2000.
6. Plato. *Res Publica* (The Republic, 360 B.C.E.). Translator, Jowett B. In: Great Books of the Western World (Hutchins RM, Editor-in-Chief). Chicago: Encyclopaedia Britannica, Inc., 1952; 295–441.
7. Aristotle. *Ethica Nicomachea* (Nicomachean Ethics, 350 B.C.E.). Translator, Ross WD. In: Great Books of the Western World (Hutchins RM, Editor-in-Chief). Chicago: Encyclopaedia Britannica, Inc., 1952; 339–444.
8. Epictetus. *Diatribai* (Discourses, circa C.E. 138). Translator, Long G. In: Great Books of the Western World (Hutchins RM, Editor-in-Chief). Chicago: Encyclopaedia Britannica, Inc., 1952; 105–252.
9. Cicero MT. *De Re Publica* (The Republic, 51 B.C.E.). Translator and Editor, Zetzel JEG. Cambridge, England: Cambridge Publishing Company, Ltd, 1995.
10. Seneca LA. *Epistulae Morales ad Lucilium* (Epistles Regarding Morals to Lucilium, C.E. 65). Latina Romono Bibliotheca, Latina Intra Text, 2006. http://info@intratext.com//.
11. Marcus Aurelius AA. *Ta eis heauton* (Meditations, C.E. 170–180). Translator, Long G. Cambridge, Massachusetts: Harvard Classics, 1862.
12. Augustine S. *De Civitate Dei* (The City of God, C.E. 426). Translator, Dods M. New York: Modem Library Paperback Classics, Random House Publishers, 2000.
13. Aquinas S.T. *Summa Theologica* (Systematic Theology, 1265–1274). Translators and Publishers, Fathers of the English Dominican Province, 1920.
14. Lucretius. *De Rerum Natura* (On the Nature of Things, 94 B.C.E.). Translator, Latham RE. Revised Edition, New York: Penguin Classics, 1994.
15. Locke J. An Essay Concerning Human Understanding (1690). Collator and Annotator, Froyer AC. In: Great Books of the Western World (Hutchins RM, Editor-in-Chief). Chicago: Encyclopaedia Britannica, Inc., 1952; 85–402.
16. Kant L. *Kritik der Reinen Vernuft* (Critique of Pure Reason, 1781). Translators and Editors, Guyer P, Wood AW. Cambridge, England: Cambridge University Press, 1998.
17. Kant L. *Kritik, der Praktischen Vernuft* (Critique of Practical Reason, 1788). Translator, Abbott JK. Cambridge, England: Cambridge University Press, 1998.
18. Kant L. *Grundlegung zur Metaphysik der Sitten* (Groundwork of Metaphysics and Morals, 1785). Translator, Abbott JK. Orchard Park, New York: Broadview Press, 2005.
19. Hobbes T. Leviathan, Or, Matter, Forme and Power of a Commonwealth Ecclesiastical and Civil (1651). In: Great Books of the Western World (Hutchins RM, Editor-in-Chief). Chicago: Encyclopaedia Britannica, Inc., 1952; 39–283.
20. Machiavelli N. The Prince (1513). Translator, Marriott WK. In: Great Books of the Western World (Hutchins RM, Editor-in-Chief). Chicago: Encyclopaedia Britannica, Inc., 1952; 1–37.

21. Bentham J. Deontology; or, The Science of Morality (Bowring J, Editor). London: Longman Publishers, Ltd., 1834.
22. Mill JS. Utilitarianism (1863). In: Great Books of the Western World (Hutchins RM, Editor-in-Chief). Chicago: Encyclopaedia Britannica, Inc., 1952; 445–76.
23. Weber M. *Politik als Beruf* (Essays in Sociology, 1919). Translators, Gerth HH and Mills CW. Oxford, England: Oxford University Press, 1946.
24. Dewey J. The study of ethics: a syllabus. Ann Arbor, Michigan: Register Publishing Co., 1894.
25. Ross WO. The right and the good. Oxford, England: Clarendon Press, 1930.
26. Editorial Board. The Nuremberg code. J Am Med Assoc. 1996;276:1691.
27. Editorial Board. World Medical Association. Declaration of Helsinki. J Am Med Assoc. 1997;277:925–6.
28. National Commission for the Protection of Human Subjects of Biomedical and Behavioral Research. The Belmont Report. Washington, DC: U.S. Government Printing Office, 1979.
29. Council for International Organizations of Medical Sciences (C.I.O.M.S.). International ethical guidelines for biomedical research involving human subjects. Geneva, Switzerland: C.I.O.M.S, 1993.
30. Levine RJ. Ethics and regulations of clinical research. Second Edition, New Haven, Connecticut: Yale University Press, 1988.
31. Emanuel EJ, Wendler D, Grady C. What makes clinical research ethical? J Am Med Assoc. 2000;283:2701–11.
32. William of Ockham. *Exposito Aurea et Admodum Utilis Super Artem Veterem Aristotelis*, (1323). Bologna, Italy: Benedictus Hectoris, 1496.
33. Taylor HJ. The story of the 4-way test. Rotary International, 1954–1955.
34. President's Commission for the Study of Ethical Problems in Medicine and Biomedical and Behavioral Research. Screening and Counseling for Genetic Conditions: A Report on the Ethical, Social, and Legal Implications of Genetic Screening, Counseling, and Education Programs. Washington, DC: U.S. Government Printing Office, 1983.
35. Hippocrates. Oath. Hippocratic Writings (400 B.C.E.). Translator, Adams F. In: Great Books of the Western World (Hutchins RM, Editor-in-Chief). Chicago: Encyclopaedia Britannica, Inc., 1952; xiii.
36. Wertz DC, Fletcher JC, Berg K. Review of Ethical Issues in Medical Genetics, Report of Consultants to WHO. Human Genetics Programme. Management of Noncommunicable Diseases. Geneva, Switzerland: World Health Organization, 2003.
37. American Society of Human Genetics Board of Directors, American College of Medical Genetics Board of Directors. Points to consider: ethical, legal and psychosocial implications of genetic testing in children and adolescents. Am J Hum Genet. 1995;57:1233–41.
38. Wertz DC, Fanos JH, Reilly PR. Genetic testing for children and adolescents: who decides? J Am Med Assoc. 1994;272(11):875–81.
39. Duncan RE, Belmett F, Martin BD. Refusing to provide a prenatal test: can it ever be ethical? Br Med J. 2006;333:1066–8.
40. Clinical Genetics Society. The genetic testing of children. Working Party of the Clinical Genetics Society (UK). J Med Genet. 1994;31:785–97.
41. Human Genetics Society of Australia. Predictive testing in children and adolescents (version 2, April 2005). http://www.hgsa.com.au//.
42. Offit K, Kohut K, Clagett B, et al. Cancer genetic testing and assisted reproduction. J Clin Reprod. 2006;24(29):4775–82.
43. Ethics Committee Report, American Society for Reproductive Medicine. Fertility preservation and reproduction in cancer patients. Fertil Steril. 2005;83(6):1622–8.
44. Verlinsky Y, Cohen J, Santiago M, et al. Over a decade of experience with preimplantation genetic diagnosis: a multicenter report. Fertil Steril. 2004;82(2):292–4.
45. Williams C, Ehrich K, Farsides B, et al. Facilitating choice, framing choice: staff views on widening the scope of preimplantation genetics diagnosis in the UK. Soc Sci Med. 2007;65(6):1094–1105.

46. Oftit K, Sagi M, Hurley K. Preimplantation genetic diagnosis for cancer syndromes: a new challenge for preventive medicine. J Am Med Assoc. 2006;296(22):2727–2730.
47. Verlinsky Y, Rechitsky S, Schoolcraft W, et al. Preimplantation diagnosis for Fanconi anemia combined with HLA matching. J Am Med Assoc. 2001;285:3130–3.
48. Kevles DJ. In the name of eugenics: genetics and the uses of human heredity. Cambridge, Massachusetts: Harvard University Press, 1985; 1995.
49. Stein AM. Eugenic nation: faults and frontiers of better breeding in modern America. Berkeley, California: University of California Press, 2005.
50. Lombardo PA. Three Generations, No Imbeciles: Virginia Eugenics and Buck v. Bell. Sixth Annual Kenneth R. Crispell Memorial History Lecture, Health Sciences Library, University of Virginia, Charlottesville, Virginia, April 23, 2002. http://www.healthsystem.virginia.edu//.
51. Shute N. Unraveling your DNA's secrets. US News & World Report. January 8, 2007; 51–58.
52. The Hastings Center, College of Physicians and Surgeons/Columbia University. Genetic Dilemmas in Primary Care. http://www.geneticdilemmas.org//.
53. Pope A. Essay on man (1733–1734). In: Selected Works of Alexander Pope. New York: Modern Library, Random House Publishers, 1948.

Chapter 4
Hereditary Breast Cancer Syndromes

Alfredo A. Santillan, Jeffrey M. Farma, Ramona Hagmaier, Charles E. Cox, and Adam I. Riker

Introduction

Breast cancer represents a major public health problem in the world. According to the GLOBOCAN database, breast cancer is the second most common cancer in the world and the most common cancer among women, accounting for an estimated 1,152,161 new cases each year and 411,093 cancer deaths per year (Fig. 4.1) [1]. In the United States, breast cancer is the second leading cause of cancer death among women after lung cancer [2]. Recent trends in the incidence of female breast cancer have shown a sharp decrease during the period of 1999–2003. This can be partly explained by the increased utilization of screening mammography, better technologies that increase the sensitivity of detection suspicious abnormalities, and an overall reduction in the use of hormone replacement therapy (Fig. 4.2) [3]. Despite this recent decrease in breast cancer incidence, it is estimated that in the year 2007, more than 178,480 women will be diagnosed with breast cancer in the United States, with approximately 40,460 women dying from this disease. Of these, about 5–10% of the total breast cancer burden will be hereditary, having affected approximately 8,924–17,848 patients during 2007 [2].

Inherited or hereditary breast cancer refers to breast cancer associated with a known or suspected high-penetrance or low-to-moderate gene mutation, which are inherited in an autosomal-dominant fashion [4]. All forms of hereditary breast cancer seem to show significant genotypic and phenotypic heterogeneity, and it is therefore important to note the particular breast cancer-associated syndrome relating to a particular family with its associated mutation (Table 4.1). Additionally, 15–20% of the newly diagnosed breast cancer patients will report a positive family history and will be loosely referred to as having a "familial breast cancer." This is

A.A. Santillan (✉)
Division of Surgical Oncology, Department of Surgery Cancer Therapy and Research Center, University of Texas Health Science Center at San Antonio, 78229, San Antonio, TX, USA
e-mail: santillangom@uthscsa.edu

C.N. Ellis (ed.), *Inherited Cancer Syndromes: Current Clinical Management*,
DOI 10.1007/978-1-4419-6821-0_4, © Springer Science+Business Media, LLC 2011

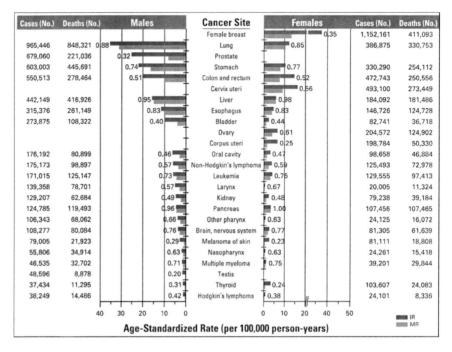

Cases (No.)	Deaths (No.)	Males		Cancer Site	Females		Cases (No.)	Deaths (No.)
				Female breast		0.35	1,152,161	411,093
965,446	848,321	0.88		Lung	0.85		386,875	330,753
679,060	221,036	0.32		Prostate				
603,003	445,691	0.74		Stomach	0.77		330,290	254,112
550,513	278,464	0.51		Colon and rectum	0.52		472,743	250,556
				Cervix uteri	0.56		493,100	273,449
442,149	416,926	0.95		Liver	0.98		184,092	181,486
315,376	261,149	0.83		Esophagus	0.83		146,726	124,728
273,875	108,322	0.40		Bladder	0.44		82,741	36,718
				Ovary	0.61		204,572	124,902
				Corpus uteri	0.25		198,784	50,330
176,192	80,899	0.46		Oral cavity	0.47		98,658	46,884
175,173	98,897	0.57		Non-Hodgkin's lymphoma	0.59		125,493	72,978
171,015	125,147	0.73		Leukemia	0.76		129,555	97,413
139,358	78,701	0.57		Larynx	0.67		20,005	11,324
129,207	62,684	0.49		Kidney	0.48		79,238	39,184
124,785	119,493	0.96		Pancreas	1.00		107,456	107,465
106,343	68,062	0.66		Other pharynx	0.63		24,125	16,072
108,277	80,084	0.76		Brain, nervous system	0.77		81,305	61,639
79,005	21,923	0.29		Melanoma of skin	0.23		81,111	18,808
55,806	34,914	0.63		Nasopharynx	0.63		24,261	15,418
46,535	32,702	0.71		Multiple myeloma	0.75		39,201	29,844
48,596	8,878	0.20		Testis				
37,434	11,295	0.31		Thyroid	0.24		103,607	24,083
38,249	14,486	0.42		Hodgkin's lymphoma	0.38		24,101	8,336

40   30   20   10   0   0   10   20   40   50

Age-Standardized Rate (per 100,000 person-years)

■ IR
■ MR

Fig. 4.1 Worldwide annual number of cases and cancer deaths, incidence rates (IRs), mortality rates (MRs), and mortality-to-incidence rate ratios (MR:IR; adjacent to bars) according to cancer site and sex (1993–2001) (adapted with permission from Kamangar F, Dores GM, Anderson WF. Patterns of cancer incidence, mortality, and prevalence across five continents: defining priorities to reduce cancer disparities in different geographic regions of the world. J Clin Oncol 2006;24:2137–2150)

somewhat of a crude classification system which is often defined as the index patient with breast cancer. This may also include one or more of her first- and/or second-degree relatives manifesting breast cancer. It is estimated that all the currently known breast cancer susceptibility genes account for less than 25% of the familial aggregation of breast cancer [4]. Therefore, it is important to understand that not all women with familial breast cancer will have a hereditary susceptibility to developing breast cancer [5–7].

Familial breast cancer tends to have a later age of onset and affects fewer persons in the family than does the hereditary breast cancer. Several non-genetic factors can lead to familial clustering of breast cancer, including: (1) a large family in which many women reach an older age (breast cancer develops in about 12% of women who live to age 90), with chance alone also contributing to the development of breast cancer; (2) an extended family living in the same geographic location with exposure to similar environmental carcinogens; (3) culturally motivated behavior that may alter risk factor profiles such as age at first live birth and breastfeeding practices; and (4) socioeconomic influences that might result in differing dietary exposures and the access to healthcare facilities and physicians. Finally, there are

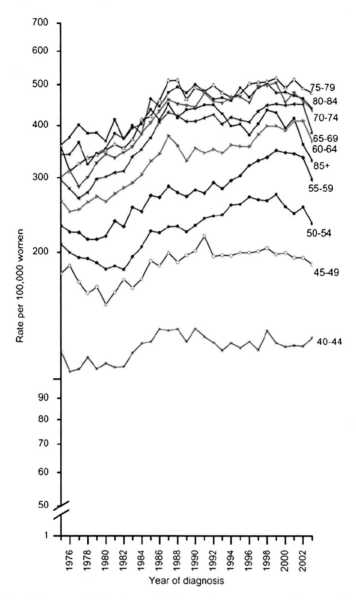

Fig. 4.2 Trends in age-specific breast cancer incidence rates among women 40 years old and above, 1975–2003 (adapted with permission from Jemal A, Ward E, Thun MJ. Recent trends in breast cancer incidence rates by age and tumor characteristics among U.S. women. Breast Cancer Res 2007;9:R28)

multiple other unclassified genetic factors that may indirectly influence the development of breast cancer in any individual, many of which can be shared among genetically similar members of an extended family [8]. The remainder of the incident cases of breast cancer are commonly classified as "sporadic," and represent

Table 4.1 Genes known to be associated with a hereditary predisposition to breast cancer

Gene	Chromosome site	Syndrome	Incidence in hereditary breast cancer (%)
BRCA1	17q21	Hereditary breast ovarian cancer	~45
BRCA2	13q12–13	Hereditary breast ovarian cancer	~35
P53	17p13.1	Li-Fraumeni	~1
PTEN	10q22–23	Cowden's disease, Bannayan-Riley-Ruvalcaba, Proteus, Proteus-like syndrome	<1
STK11/LKB1	19p13.3	Peutz-Jeghers	<1
CDH1		Hereditary diffuse gastric carcinoma	<1
ATM	11q22–23	Ataxia-telangiectasia	<1
CHEK2	22q12.1	Li-Fraumeni variant, Ataxia-telangiectasia	<1
BRIP1	17q22–24	Fanconi's anemia	<1
PALB2	16p12.1	None known	<1

those patients who lack any significant family history of breast cancer throughout their family pedigree (Table 4.2).

Recent advances in molecular biology and the many discoveries in the human genome have revealed a number of germline mutations that have been shown to predispose one to breast cancer. Hereditary breast cancer is no longer considered a rare disease, but rather it is a topic of considerable interest to both physicians and the general public. The incidence of hereditary breast cancer among women in 2007 will roughly equal the incidence in total of several other cancers, such as the pancreas, rectum, bladder, kidney, leukemia, and oral/pharyngeal cancers [2]. It is now possible to offer predictive DNA testing to individuals with a high risk of harboring a susceptible gene. The increased awareness of cancer risk combined with the availability of genetic testing for breast cancer has made hereditary breast cancer a topic of extreme relevance among clinicians involved in breast cancer care. Furthermore, the considerable research involved with hereditary breast cancer has provided new insights into the etiology of breast cancer, allowing for the rapid translation of such discoveries into diagnostic tests for earlier diagnosis, prognostic stratification, and better treatment strategies for those patients with breast cancer.

Hereditary Breast and Ovarian Cancer Syndrome

Susceptible Genes

A germline mutation in the BRCA1 or BRCA2 gene is the most commonly detectable cause of a hereditable risk of breast cancer. Both genes normally function as tumor suppressor genes, with the aberrant function of these genes responsible for

Table 4.2 Characteristics of hereditary, familial, and sporadic breast cancer syndromes

	Characteristics
Hereditary cancer	• Autosomal-dominant transmission of specific cancer type(s) • Earlier age of onset of cancer than is typical • Multiple primary cancers in an individual • Clustering of rare cancers • Bilateral or multifocal cancers • First-degree relatives of mutation carriers are at 50% risk to have the same mutation • Incomplete penetrance and variable expressivity, such that obligate carriers of the family mutation may be cancer-free and the age of diagnosis of cancer among relatives will vary • Those who do not have the familial mutation have the general population risk for cancer
Familial cancer	• More cases of a specific type(s) of cancer within a family than statistically expected, but no specific pattern of inheritance • Age of onset variable • May result from chance clustering of sporadic cases • May result from common genetic background, similar environment and/or lifestyle factors • Does not usually exhibit classical features of hereditary cancer syndromes
Sporadic cancer	• Cancers in the family are likely due to nonhereditary causes • Typical age of onset • Even if there is more than one case in the family, there is no particular pattern of inheritance • Very low likelihood that genetic susceptibility testing will reveal a mutation; testing will likely not provide additional information about cancer risk

Source: Adapted with permission from Berliner JL, Fay AM. Risk assessment and genetic counseling for hereditary breast and ovarian cancer: recommendations of the National Society of Genetic Counselors. J Genet Counsel 2007;16:241–260

an estimated 5–15% of all newly diagnosed breast cancers. However, only about 40–50% of families with multiple cases of female breast cancer, with no known cases of ovarian or male breast cancer, are definitively linked to these genes. In contrast, the combination of breast and ovarian cancer within families is highly correlated with *BRCA1* and *BRCA2* germline mutations, often referred to as the hereditary breast and ovarian cancer syndrome (HBOC). Most known genetic mutations are inherited in an autosomal dominant fashion with high penetrance, with the risk equal for males and females.

Defining the penetrance associated with these germline mutations may be confounded by the method of family ascertainment in the study and by undefined superimposed variations in genetic or environmental risks. Furthermore, the degree of penetrance may vary according to the specific gene and locus that is mutated [9]. Another contributor to the variation in the rates of penetrance is related to whether the female has undergone oophorectomy, which has been shown to contribute a relative protection against the development of breast cancer [10]. A reliable estimate of penetrance is crucial for the proper counseling and decision making for patients with the HBOC syndrome. For instance, women who carry these *BRCA1* and *BRCA2* mutations have an estimated lifetime breast cancer risk between 60 and 85%, with a lifetime ovarian cancer risk between 26 and 54% for *BRCA1*, and between 10 and 23% for *BRCA2* [11–13]. However, these risks are derived from populations of women that are closely followed in high-risk clinics, and, thus, are somewhat biased toward a slightly higher incidence of genetic breast cancer. In contrast, population-based studies suggest a lower lifetime overall risk of ~40–50% for the development of genetic breast cancer [14–17].

A recent meta-analysis was performed to help genetic counselors and clinicians estimate the overall genetic risk based on a comprehensive set of ten studies conducted in high-risk clinics and population-based settings [18]. The cumulative breast cancer risk for *BRCA1* and *BRCA2* mutation carriers at age 70 years was found to be 57% (95% confidence interval, 47–66%) and 49% (95% confidence interval, 40–57%), respectively. The ovarian cancer risk association with the *BRCA1* gene was found to be higher compared to the *BRCA2* gene, with a cumulative cancer risk for ovarian cancer for *BRCA1* carriers of 40% (95% confidence interval, 35–46%) compared to 18% (95% confidence intervals, 13–23%) among *BRCA2* carriers. Furthermore, unlike male carriers of *BRCA1* mutations who do not have a known associated risk of breast cancer, men with germline mutations in *BRCA2* have an estimated 6% lifetime breast cancer risk, representing a 100-fold increase over the general male population [19]. Thus, it is important for those clinicians counseling known patients whom carry a mutation for either breast or ovarian cancer to not solely focus on the single point estimates, but instead provide an overall range of risk based upon all of the available data (Table 4.3).

The exact molecular mechanism by which a *BRCA* mutation predisposes a patient to the development of cancer is not fully understood. Recent data suggest that a germline mutation occurs within the BRCA gene, representing the first "hit" of Knudsen's two-hit model of tumorigenesis [20]. These mutations are thought to interfere with the DNA repair function of the normal gene, resulting in the accumulation of chromosomal abnormalities and a propensity to develop malignancy. If the second allele of the gene develops a point mutation or other defect, the stage is then set for the development of cancer in the future [20].

BRCA1

BRCA1 is located on chromosome 17q, spanning a genomic region of about 100 kb of DNA, and containing a total of 24 coding exons. The full-length mRNA is 7.8 kb and encodes a protein of 1,863 amino acids in humans. Approximately 45% of all hereditary breast cancer-prone families, including those characterized as HBOC, are due to mutations of the *BRCA1* gene, whereas a slightly lower percentage is due to *BRCA2* mutations [12, 21, 22]. The *BRCA1* was first isolated in 1990 and subsequently cloned in 1994 [23, 24]. Since this discovery, hundreds of different mutations have been identified [25]. Initially, eight disease-associated mutations were

Table 4.3 Predicted mean cancer risk to currently unaffected *BRCA1/2* mutation carriers

Risk (%) of developing cancer by age

Current age	30 Years Mean	95% CI	40 Years Mean	95% CI	50 Years Mean	95% CI	60 Years Mean	95% CI	70 Years Mean	95% CI
Breast cancer: *BRCA1*										
20 years	1.8	1.4–2.2	12	9.5–14	29	24–35	44	37–52	54	46–63
30 years			10	8.2–13	28	23–34	44	36–52	54	45–63
40 years					20	16–25	38	31–45	49	41–58
50 years							22	18–27	37	30–44
60 years									19	15–24
Breast cancer: *BRCA2*										
20 years	1	0.8–1.4	7.5	5.8–9.8	21	17–26	35	28–42	45	38–53
30 years			6.6	5.1–8.6	20	16–26	35	28–42	45	38–53
40 years					15	12–19	30	24–36	42	34–49
50 years							18	15–22	32	26–38
60 years									17	14–20
Ovarian cancer: *BRCA1*										
20 years	1	0.7–1.8	3.2	2.3–5.1	9.5	7.3–13	23	18–28	39	34–44
30 years			2.2	1.6–3.4	8.7	6.7–12	22	18–27	39	34–43
40 years					6.7	5.2–8.9	20	17–24	38	33–41
50 years							15	12–17	34	29–36
60 years									22	20–23
Ovarian cancer: *BRCA2*										
20 years	0.19	0.1–0.05	0.7	0.4–1.5	2.6	1.5–4.5	7.5	2.1–11	16	12–20
30 years			0.5	0.3–1	2.4	1.5–4.2	7.4	5.1–11	16	12–20
40 years					1.9	1.2–3.2	7	4.8–10	16	12–20
50 years							5.2	3.7–7.2	14	11–17
60 years									9.8	7.8–11

Source: Adapted with permission from Chen S, Parmigiani G. Meta-analysis of *BRCA1* and *BRCA2* penetrance. J Clin Oncol 2007:25:1329–1333

described within the *BRCA* gene [24, 26] followed rapidly by an increasing number of novel mutations [27–29]. Most of the mutations are either frameshift or missense mutations, but several splice acceptor and donor sites are also found to be frequently mutated.

Mutations are common in women of Ashkenazi Jewish (Eastern European) descent, in whom approximately 2.3% carry a deleterious *BRCA* mutation [15]. Between 12 and 30% of breast cancers in this ethnic group are thought to be attributable to *BRCA* mutations [16, 30–32]. Several founder mutations have been identified in *BRCA1*, representing specific genetic changes that are consistently associated with a certain disease in defined populations. The two most common mutations are 185delAG and 5382insC, which account for approximately 10% of all the mutations seen in *BRCA1* [33]. These two mutations occur at a tenfold higher frequency in the Ashkenazi Jewish population compared to non-Jewish Caucasians [15, 34]. The carrier frequency of the 185delAG mutation in Ashkenazi Jews is approximately 1%, with the 5382insC mutation accounting for almost all of the known *BRCA1* mutations in this population [35, 36]. Analysis of germline mutations in Jewish and non-Jewish women with early-onset breast cancer indicates that approximately 20% of Jewish women who develop breast cancer before the age of 40 carry the 185delAG mutation [30, 37].

Early attempts to create animal models to further study *BRCA1* homozygous deletions and mutation associated breast cancer have not been very successful, mostly due the fact that *BRCA1* deficiency invariably results in embryonic lethality secondarily to elevated cell death and growth retardation [38, 39]. The normal *BRCA1* protein is involved in DNA repair mechanisms important for homologous recombination, transcriptional regulation, cell cycle control, and ubiquitination [40]. Specifically, the *BRCA1* protein has been shown to facilitate repair of DNA double-strand breaks caused by ionizing radiation and to inhibit S-phase progression via the dephosphorylation of the retinoblastoma (Rb) protein, E2F binding, and possibly CDK2 gene repression [41].

Mutations of the *BRCA1* gene can also directly inhibit *p53* transcription, whereas other *BRCA1* mutations function as negative inhibitors of *p53*. One key function of *p53* is G1 to S-phase cell cycle control. Disruption of *p53* function may allow for both the persistence of cells with DNA mutations and the inhibition of damaged cells from undergoing apoptosis. Normal *BRCA1* protein function has also been associated with c-Myc repression [42]. *BRCA1* interacts directly or indirectly with numerous cellular molecules, including tumor suppressors, oncogenes, DNA damage repair proteins, cell cycle regulators, transcriptional activators, and repressors [43–55]. Consistent with this extensive pattern of interaction, loss-of-function mutations of *BRCA1* result in pleotrophic phenotypes, leading to growth retardation, increased apoptosis, defective mechanisms of DNA repair, abnormal centrosome duplication, defective G_2/M cell cycle regulation, and chromosomal damage [56–58]. These phenotypes do not seem to be compatible with the normal tumor suppressor functions assigned to *BRCA1*, and it has been proposed that such mutations do not directly result in tumor formation, but instead, cause overall genetic instability that results in a high subsequent risk of malignant transformation (Fig. 4.3) [59].

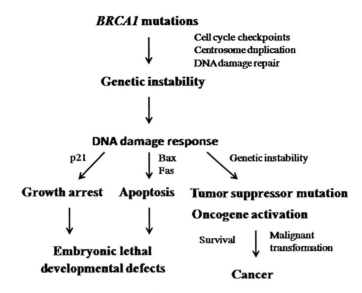

Fig. 4.3 A model illustrating connections among cell cycle checkpoints, centrosome duplication, DNA damage repair, genetic instability, DNA damage response, developmental abnormalities, and tumorigenesis caused by *BRCA1* deficiency (adapted with permission from Deng C. *BRCA1*: cell cycle checkpoint, genetic instability, DNA damage response and cancer evolution. Nucleic Acids Res 2006;34:1416–1426)

BRCA2

The *BRCA2* gene is located on chromosome 13q12–13 and spans a genomic region of about 70 kb of DNA. The 11.2-kb coding region contains 26 coding exons and encodes a protein comprised of 3,418 amino acids. The *BRCA2* gene bears no homology to any previously described gene, and the protein contains no previously defined functional domains. The biologic function of *BRCA2* is not well defined, but, like *BRCA1*, it is thought to play a role in the repair of DNA damage. Specifically, this protein has been shown to bind Rad51, important for meiotic and mitotic recombination and double-strand break repairs. *BRCA2* has also been associated with proliferating nuclear cell antigen (PCNA) which is also involved in DNA repair and replication [42, 60]. *BRCA2* messenger RNA is expressed at high levels in the late G1 and S phases of the cell cycle, with the cell kinetics of *BRCA2* protein regulation similar to that of *BRCA1* protein [61]. Furthermore, the over-expression of *BRCA2* has also been found to repress *p53* [42].

The mutational spectrum of *BRCA2* is not as well established as that of *BRCA1*. There have been over 250 *BRCA2* mutations identified, with many resulting in truncated protein products, missense mutations, and over-expression of the *BRCA2* protein [62–72]. Mutations can be found to be spread fairly uniformly throughout the gene, without well-defined hot spots. A number of founder mutations have also been identified in *BRCA2*, with the 6174delT mutation found in Ashekanzi Jews having a prevalence of 1.2% [73]. Another *BRCA2* founder mutation, 999del5, has been observed in Icelandic and Finnish populations [74, 75]. The Icelandic and Finnish mutation carriers share a common haplotype that covers a region spanning the *BRCA2* gene, suggesting that individuals who migrated from Finland to Iceland during ancient times most likely carried this specific mutation [76].

We do not fully understand why certain *BRCA* mutations predispose one to primarily breast and ovarian cancers. Preclinical data suggest that intact *BRCA* function represents a barrier to ligand-independent transcriptional activation of the estrogen receptor, and that functional inactivation could possibly lead to altered hormonal regulation of mammary and ovarian epithelial proliferation [56, 77].

Identifying Hereditary Risk for Breast Cancer

A critical component in the management of hereditary breast cancer is being able to determine which patients are most likely to harbor gene mutations that can be identified with genetic testing. Recognition of those patients with an increased risk for the development of hereditary breast cancer is essential for providing the opportunity for primary prevention, as well as for targeting high-risk groups for earlier diagnosis and treatment. Identifying a population of patients with a hereditary risk for breast cancer is a five-step process that includes: (1) obtaining a complete family history, (2) assessing the appropriateness of genetic testing, (3) pre- and posttest counseling of the patient, (4) protection for genetic discrimination, and (5) interpreting the results of testing.

Family History

A significant family history of breast cancer markedly influences a woman's risk for developing breast cancer in the future (Table 4.4). Approximately 12% of American women are considered to have a "family history" of breast cancer by history [78]. A meta-analysis of over 74 studies worldwide found that such women have a lifetime chance of developing breast cancer that is about twofold higher than that of the general population [79]. Furthermore, between 20 and 30% of women with breast cancer have at least one relative with the disease,[6, 7] with only 5–10% having a true hereditary predisposition [80, 81]. Therefore, in order to accurately establish the diagnosis of a hereditary breast cancer syndrome, a detailed analysis of a patient's cancer history within the family is essential prior to considering formal genetic testing [82]. It is important to assess both a maternal and paternal family history, as one half of women with a *BRCA* mutation will have inherited it from their fathers. Construction of a pedigree is central to accurately estimate the risk of developing breast cancer, in addition to estimating the likelihood of carrying a high-penetrant gene mutation within the family. To construct a pedigree, one must record the type of cancer and its origin, the age of each family member when they are

Table 4.4 Risk of breast cancer according to family history

	Relative risk estimates (95% CI)
Any family history	1.9 (1.7–2.0)
Type of family history	
First degree	2.1 (2.0–2.2)
Second degree	1.5 (1.4–1.6)
Number of affected relatives	
One first degree	2.1 (2.0–2.2)
Two first degree	3.6 (2.5–5.0)
Age of affected relatives	
First degree <50 years	2.3 (2.2–2.5)
First degree >50 years	1.8 (1.6–2.0)
Type of cancer	
First degree with bilateral breast cancer	9.8 (4.0–24.9)
First degree with ovarian cancer	1.3 (0.9–1.8)

diagnosed, the age and cause of death, the presence or absence of all surgeries performed, and the ethnicity/racial background.

The importance of the pedigree is illustrated by the high prevalence of *BRCA* gene mutations among women of Ashkenazi Jewish descent. The frequency of *BRCA* mutations in the general population of most Western societies varies significantly, but is reported to be somewhere between 0.05 and 0.32 per 100 women for *BRCA1* and between 0.07 and 0.76 for *BRCA2* [83–86]. In contrast, founder mutations of *BRCA1* and *BRCA2* in the Ashkenazi Jewish population occur with a background frequency of 2.3% [15, 87]. It is estimated that between 50 and 90% of Jewish families with a strong family history of breast and ovarian cancer and 12% of Ashkenazi Jews with breast cancer harbor at least one of the founding mutations. Other ethnic groups with a high prevalence of founder mutations include families from Iceland, Poland, Sweden, and the Netherlands [88, 89]. The threshold for genetic testing should be lower in such populations where the prevalence of mutations is known to be higher compared to the general population.

In addition to racial/ethnic background, the age at cancer diagnosis is also a factor that is highly associated with the probability of finding a founding mutation, even in those individuals without a strong family history of cancer. For instance, about 20–30% of Jewish women who developed breast cancer before the age of 40 without any significant family history, and 38–60% of those with ovarian cancer diagnosed prior to age 50, harbored a founding mutation in the *BRCA1* gene [30–32, 90]. The importance of taking a good history with the construction of a family pedigree for cancer is crucial and may constitute the most cost-beneficial strategy for determining the overall risks for patients.

Cardinal features of hereditary cancer syndromes are the development of multiple cancers in the family, multiple primary tumors in an individual, a younger age of presentation, and vertical transmission. Features suggestive of HBOC and therefore *BRCA* germline mutation in an individual family include: two or more women with ovarian cancer or breast cancer before age 50, women with more than one primary cancer such as bilateral breast cancer or breast plus ovarian cancer, and evidence of vertical transmission consistent with autosomal dominant inheritance. Any woman diagnosed with breast cancer before the age of 50 or ovarian cancer at any age should be counseled about genetic cancer risks. Further inquiry should be made about any first-, second-, and third-degree relatives on either side of the family with a history of cancer. Male breast cancer at any age also suggests the possibility of HBOC. If these features are present while obtaining the family history, further discussion should ensure as to the possibility of a germline mutation in either of the *BRCA* genes.

On the other hand, clinicians will frequently encounter families with either a limited number of members or a limited family history. The variable expressivity and incomplete penetrance of susceptibility genes affect the ability to identify a pattern of hereditary breast cancer in some families. Determining the risk of harboring a susceptible germline mutation in these individuals will become exceedingly difficult, further complicated by the complexities of both environmental and genetic factors. One must use the available epidemiologic studies to assess and estimate a woman's risk of developing breast cancer, incorporating as many other risk factors that may play a role, such as the reproductive history. In contrast, if the family history is suggestive of hereditary breast cancer, risk assessment is based upon probabilistic estimates of identifying a gene mutation with the risk of developing cancer based upon the known estimates of gene penetrance.

Risk Assessment Models

The average lifetime risk of breast cancer in the United States female population at birth is 12%, or approximately one in eight women [91]. The longer a woman lives without cancer, the lower her risk of subsequently developing breast cancer. Thus, a 50-year-old woman has an 11% lifetime risk of developing breast cancer, while a 70-year-old woman has a 7% lifetime risk of developing breast cancer. Many epidemiological studies have attempted to evaluate relevant risk factors for developing breast cancer, but because these factors interact and modify risk, evaluating the actual risk conferred by multiple factors can be challenging [92–94]. Furthermore, risk factors infrequently associated with breast cancer, such as diet, oral contraceptive use, lactation, abortion history, or radiation exposure, have not been included in most risk assessment models [95–98].

An important area of ongoing research involves determining whether factors that alter breast cancer risk in the general population also affect the risk in *BRCA* mutation carriers. Breast cancer risk in the general population is closely related to reproductive history as strong candidates for modifiers of breast cancer risk in *BRCA* mutation carriers. For instance, increased parity and an earlier age of first childbirth are associated with a lower risk of developing breast cancer in the general population. This protective effect is usually restricted to women older than 40 years old.

A similar effect has been observed in the International *BRCA1/2* Carrier Cohort Study (IBCCS), where multiple full-term pregnancies were associated with a moderate reduction in the risk of breast cancer (the risk of breast cancer decreased by approximately 14% for each additional birth). The protective effect was also observed only among carriers who were older than 40 years. Furthermore, age at first full-term pregnancy and breast cancer risk differed in *BRCA1* and *BRCA2* mutation carriers. In *BRCA2* mutation carriers, full-term pregnancy before the age of 20 was associated with a lower risk of breast cancer than a later age at first pregnancy, whereas in *BRCA1* mutation carriers, a later age at first pregnancy appeared to be associated with a lower risk of breast cancer. In this cohort of patients, neither miscarriages, induced abortions, nor a history of breast feeding was associated with breast cancer risk [99, 100]. In contrast, the IBCCS group found that early age at menarche and late age at menopause were not associated with an increased breast cancer risk in *BRCA1* and *BRCA2* carriers [101]. These findings are not consistent with the results in the general population where both factors seem to be associated with an overall increased risk for the development of breast cancer. This may reflect a genuine difference in the natural history of breast cancer in *BRCA* carriers with respect to reproductive factors.

Empirical Models

Previously, there have been two risk assessment models utilized to predict the risk of developing breast cancer. From the Breast Cancer Detection Demonstration Project (BCDDP), a large mammography screening program that included 4,496 matched pair of cases, Gail et al. developed the most commonly used model in 1989 [94]. The Gail model based breast cancer risk upon defined weighted factors such as age at menarche, age at first live birth, number of previous breast biopsies, presence of atypical hyperplasia in biopsy, number of first-degree relatives with breast cancer, and race (Table 4.5). The Gail model is capable of predicting the cumulative risk of breast cancer according to the decade of life, up to the age of 90 years.

To calculate breast cancer risk with the Gail model, a woman's risk factors are translated into an overall risk score by multiplying her relative risks from several categories. The risk score is then multiplied by an adjusted population risk of breast cancer to determine the individual risk of breast cancer. A software program incorporating the Gail model is available from the National Cancer Institute at www.cancer.gov/bcrisktool. This model represents an interactive tool designed by scientists at the National Cancer Institute and the National Surgical Adjuvant Breast and Bowel Project (NSABP) to estimate a woman's risk of developing invasive breast cancer. The tool will soon be updated with more accurate risk information for African American/Black women and will be called the CARE model. The Gail model is a relatively easy and effective tool to utilize in women, having been further validated in two subsequent studies [102, 103].

Table 4.5 Relative risk estimates for the Gail model

Variable	Relative risk
I. Age at menarche (years)	
≥14	1.00
12–13	1.10
<12	1.21
II. Number of breast biopsies	
Age at counseling <50 years	
0	1.00
1	1.70
≥2	2.88
Age at counseling ≥50 years	
0	1.00
1	1.27
≥2	1.62
III. Age at first live birth	
<20 years	
Number of first-degree relatives with breast cancer	
0	1.00
1	2.61
≥2	6.80
20–24 years	
Number of first-degree relatives with breast cancer	
0	1.24
1	2.68
≥2	5.78
25–29 years	
Number of first-degree relatives with breast cancer	
0	1.55
1	2.76
≥2	4.91
≥30 years	
Number of first-degree relatives with breast cancer	
0	1.93
1	2.83
≥2	4.17
IV. Atypical hyperplasia	
No biopsies	1.00
At least one biopsy and no atypical hyperplasia	0.93
No atypical hyperplasia found and hyperplasia status unknown for at least one biopsy specimen	1.00
Atypical hyperplasia found in at least one biopsy	1.82

Although relatively good at estimating the influence of family history on breast cancer risk, the Gail model has several limitations that diminish its overall sensitivity such as the inclusion of a non-biologic variable (number of breast biopsies) and the exclusion of a more thorough and extensive family history. For instance, it does not take into account the risk of individuals who have second-degree relatives diagnosed with breast cancer or relatives diagnosed with ovarian cancer. It also excludes the age of diagnosis of relatives with breast or ovarian cancer. This notable omission of relevant data derived from the family history tend to lead to a sizable underestimation of true risk, further shown with those individuals having a history of lobular or ductal carcinoma in situ. To the contrary, the Gail model may overestimate the risk in women with non-proliferative disease of the breast.

In a modification of the original model, referred to as the Gail model 2, age-specific invasive breast cancer rates for Caucasian women from the Surveillance Epidemiology and End Results (SEER) database were substituted for the prior breast cancer incidences rates derived from BCDDP [104]. Subsequent validation studies confirmed the validity of this model in both US and non-US populations [105, 106]. Additional refinements to the Gail model, such as the inclusion of breast density at the time of screening mammography, may improve the ability to predict the absolute risk of developing invasive breast cancer in individual women [107, 108]. Indeed, the density of the breast tissue is known to be a significant risk factor associated with increased breast cancer risk in the general population as well as in those found to be carriers of either the *BRCA1* and *BRCA2* mutations [109].

Another risk assessment model was developed in 1994 by Claus et al. based upon data gathered from the Cancer and Steroid Hormone Study (CASH), which was a large, population-based, case–control study evaluating the impact of oral contraceptives on the risk of breast cancer [110]. This model was developed from the recognized prevalence of high-penetrant genes for susceptibility to breast cancer. As compared to the Gail model, the Claus model incorporates more extensive information about family history, but excludes other risk factors. On the basis of knowledge of first- and second-degree relatives with breast cancer and their age at diagnosis, the Claus model provides individual estimates of breast cancer risk according to decade, over a range of 29–79 years of age. This model was developed prior to the identification of the significance of the *BRCA* genes and is therefore based solely upon the possibility that a rare, as yet identified autosomal-dominant allele is possibly segregating within family members. Since the identification and cloning of the *BRCA* gene mutations, the utility of this model for women with a strong family history is questionable, with the probabilistic models likely to be more useful to predict if a woman harbors a susceptible mutation within these genes.

Risk estimates calculated by different models may vary; a factor that further complicates the utility of quantitative risk thresholds for making screening recommendations [111]. Most of the models have been incompletely validated, and their usefulness in non-Caucasian women and non-US populations is somewhat limited. Analyses of more heterogeneous contemporary databases suggest that there are significant age-related racial differences that may impact the calculated overall breast cancer risk. For instance, the cumulative lifetime risk for developing breast cancer among Caucasian women with at least one affected first-degree relative is 22% compared to 15% among blacks, with the difference even more pronounced as the number of affected relatives increased [112]. Thus, a degree of caution must be maintained as one attempts to interpret the degree of overall risk, no matter which model is being utilized. The limitations of each model however is overcome by the ease of obtaining this information that subsequently can be extremely useful in discussing overall risk and strategies to be utilized as a result.

Probabilistic Models

Certain models that estimate breast cancer risk are able to incorporate a Bayesian predictive algorithm for the likelihood that a woman carries a *BRCA1* or *BRCA2* mutation. These probabilistic models have been developed to assist clinicians in counseling women with a strong family or personal history of breast cancer. Bayesian modeling thus incorporates the probability that a female carries a deleterious mutation (pretest mutation probability) with the probability that a mutation will be found if she is genotyped (dependent upon the accuracy of mutation testing). With the increasing demand for an accurate assessment of the family history highlighting cancer within individual family members, numerous statistical models have been developed to estimate mutation probabilities (Table 4.6) [13, 113–126]. These models use different statistical methods, source populations, pedigree features, and predicted outcomes. Models currently used in counseling about genetic testing are included in materials distributed to women who are considering genetic testing, with some used for determining the eligibility for screening and prevention studies [127]. Mutational probability thresholds for referral were used in the past and they are still used sometimes for insurance coverage purposes [128]. However, current established guidelines no longer recommend this practice [129, 130].

BRCAPro, a computer model initially developed by Berry et al. in 1997, is one of the most commonly used probabilistic models today [117]. This model considers the structure of the family's pedigree, including both affected and unaffected family members, in estimating the probability of having a mutation in *BRCA1* or *BRCA2*. Additionally, it provides data regarding the age at initial diagnosis of breast or ovarian cancer, presence of bilateral breast cancer, male breast cancer, and Ashkenazi heritage. The model is based on prevalence, penetrance, and mutation frequency data derived from persons who have had *BRCA* mutation analysis. It also has limitations due to a lack of recognition of other risk factors besides family history and is somewhat more difficult to gather essential information as it requires information on all unaffected first- and second-degree relatives. The BRCAPro has yet to be validated in non-Caucasians populations, with only a few studies utilizing the BRCAPro model in African Americans and Hispanic populations. These smaller studies however have yielded some promising results that appear to perform equally well compared to Caucasian populations [131, 132].

A recent study evaluated the validity of seven common probabilistic methods in high-risk and population-based centers, including the BRCAPro model [127]. Comparisons across populations indicate a decrease in specificity and an increase in sensitivity as the analysis moves from population-based to high-risk studies. The concordance between predictions and test results was high in model-based mutation probabilities. However, relying solely upon model probabilities to decide about referral for genetic testing can be fraught with both false-positive and false-negative

Table 4.6 Risk models for estimating the likelihood of carrying a *BRCA1/2* mutation

Model	Characteristics	Limitations
Couch (Couch et al. [114])	Probability of detecting a *BRCA1* mutation on the basis of average age of breast cancer onset in the family, the presence of ovarian cancer, and the presence of breast and ovarian cancer in the same person. Probabilities are separated for those of Ashkenazi Jewish and non-Ashkenazi descent	Study is based on families with an average of four affected relatives (must have ≥2), which may not be helpful for smaller families or those with fewer affected members. Does not provide risk estimates for *BRCA2* and does not account for bilateral or male breast cancers. Not applicable for families with ovarian cancer only. Further calculations are needed for unaffected relatives
Myriad II (Frank et al. [121])	Provides estimation of mutation prevalence in Ashkenazi and non-Ashkenazi Jewish individuals. Incorporates those with breast and/or ovarian cancer, and separates those with breast cancer diagnosed before the age of 50 and at or after 50	May overestimate probabilities for women who have only one affected relative versus those with larger family histories. May underestimate probabilities in families with early onset breast cancer
Myriad prevalence tables	Very similar to Myriad II, and incorporates male breast cancers	Data obtained from laboratory requisition forms have not been independently verified. Proband and family history information based on that listed on the form by the clinician
BRCAPro (Berry et al., Euhus et al., and Parmigiani et al. [116, 117, 312])	Modeled probabilities base on family history of breast and ovarian cancer in first and second-degree relatives and cancer rates in *BRCA* mutation carriers derived from previous studies. Incorporates client's age and number and ages of unaffected relatives. Incorporates all affected and unaffected first and second-degree relatives, bilateral breast cancer, and Ashkenazi Jewish ancestry. Age of onset and age of unaffected relatives are considered, as are breast, ovarian, and male breast cancers. Performs slightly better in non-Ashkenazi individuals	Assumes that *BRCA1* and *BRCA2* are the only predisposition genes for breast cancer. May overestimate the probability of a mutation in families with bilateral breast cancer and underestimate risk in families with early-onset breast cancer. Does not include information on multiple marriages or extended family history

(continued)

Table 4.6 (continued)

Model	Characteristics	Limitations
Manchester (Evans et al. [124, 311])	The most sensitive model in predicting mutations in both *BRCA* genes, although works better for *BRCA2*. Outperforms Myriad II and BRCAPro with better overall prediction of the number of mutations. Incorporates pancreatic cancer. Takes minimal time and does not require computer data input	May need modification to include pathology data to calculate whether to screen for *BRCA1*. Results in over-referral for genetic testing. Was developed from non-Ashkenazi Jewish families and affected probands
BOADICEA (Breast and ovarian analysis of disease incidence and carrier estimation algorithm) (Barcenas et al. [310])	Susceptibility to *BRCA1/2* is examined along with polygenic component reflecting joint effects of multiple genes with small effects on breast cancer risk. Includes extended family data. Performs better than other models in Ashkenazi Jewish families. Slightly better results with extended family history information than with limiting information to second-degree relatives. Performs as well as BRCAPro when applied to data from first and second-degree relatives	May underestimate the observed risk at low estimated probabilities and overestimate it at higher probabilities. Does not account for male breast cancer, double primary breast or bilateral breast cancers

Source: Adapted with permission from Berliner JL, Fay AM. Risk assessment and genetic counseling for hereditary breast and ovarian cancer: recommendations of the National Society of Genetic Counselors. J Genet Counsel 2007;16:241–260

results. Therefore, decisions about genetic testing and prevention should reflect a broader range of factors, of which carrier probabilities are but one [130, 133]. Finally, a limitation of probabilistic models is that they tend to underestimate the risk of mutation probability in families with only a limited number of informative relatives in either the maternal or paternal line [134].

A recent computerized program termed CancerGene has been developed to overcome some of these limitations. The program incorporates five probabilistic models (including BRCAPro) to assess the probability that an individual is a *BRCA* gene mutation carrier. It constructs a pedigree from the family history and incorporates other models to assess breast cancer probabilities, such as the Gail and Claus models. The CancerGene model is available for download at http://www4.utsouthwestern.edu/breasthealth/cagene.

Genetic Counseling

Genetic testing for breast and ovarian cancer should be thoroughly discussed in the context of proper patient education and counseling. This includes both pre- and post-test genetic counseling, which is critical due to the complexities and implications associated with either a positive or negative result. The downstream effects have important implications for subsequent treatment recommendations in addition to the potential psychosocial ramifications of test results [130]. Genetic testing for breast and ovarian cancer susceptibility is performed only with an individual's informed consent, including signing of a document to certify that informed consent was obtained. The review and signing of the informed consent form establish that appropriate discussion with the patient has taken place, and that the patient fully understands the risks, benefits, and limitations of genetic testing. Unlike other diagnostic tests, the identification of a possible hereditary susceptibility to breast cancer has significant implications not only for the individual being tested, but also for the individual's relatives. Appropriate counseling includes discussing the basic principles of hereditary cancer susceptibility, reviewing the patient's complete family cancer history, assessing the risk of cancer, and explaining how testing helps characterize the patient's risks and the implications of a positive, negative, or indeterminate result. In addition to addressing genetic and medical issues, it is also important to discuss the psychosocial aspects of testing with patients. In particular, it is important to include the risk of misattributed paternity in the informed consent process for counseling.

A recent meta-analysis demonstrated that genetic counseling significantly improved a patient knowledge of genetics, and the accuracy of perceived risk, but it did not significantly impact upon general anxiety or cancer-specific concerns [135]. It is important to clearly discuss the impact of a positive test for other family members as well, focusing the discussion in terms that can be understood by all members of the family involved. This can be challenging, because many patients assume that they often have a much higher risk based upon personal family experiences with cancer. It is sometimes difficult to differentiate and clearly explain the differences between probability and overall risk and it is recommended that the patient and family members seek out the expertise of a genetic counselor if available. However, this may be difficult for many areas of the United States where such expertise may not be immediately available.

Given the complexities and challenges inherent in the decision to undergo genetic testing, it is not surprising that many high-risk women choose not to learn more about their genetic status, even after counseling. In several studies, only about 50% of women followed in high risk cancer clinics decided to be tested for a *BRCA* mutation [136–138]. The reasons most commonly given for declining genetic testing are lack of health insurance, possible insurance discrimination, potential effects on self and family, and concerns about test accuracy [129, 136].

Genetic Discrimination

Concerns have been raised that the identification of an individual with hereditary breast or ovarian cancer can interfere with access to affordable health insurance, have negative effects on employment, and lead to inadequate protection of privacy. This concern refers to discrimination directed against an individual or family based solely on an apparent or perceived genetic variation from normal human genotype [139]. Despite these concerns, there is no evidence to date that genetic discrimination is an emerging problem [140, 141]. In fact, there are only rare cases whereby health insurers have inquired about patient's pre-symptomatic genetic testing results in their underwriting decisions [141].

Privacy laws regarding confidentiality of health information should provide a system that is strong enough to reassure patients that genetic test results will not be used to discriminate against them. The Health Insurance Portability and Accountability Act of 1996 (HIPPA) made it illegal in the United States for group health plans to consider genetic information a pre-existing condition or use it to deny or limit coverage. However, it fails to extend these protections to individuals who are purchasing coverage in the individual market, and does not limit the ability of insurers to collect or require genetic information for those applying for health insurance. In the year 2000, an executive order prohibited discrimination of federal employees based upon genetic information, however, there are currently no federal laws or statutes in place that prohibit or ban genetic discrimination among the general population. The Genetic Information Nondiscrimination Act, which would prohibit health insurers and employers from asking or requiring a person to take a genetic test and from using genetic test information in setting insurance rates or making employment decisions, was originally introduced as new legislation in 2003, and was passed in 2007 [142]. Most states have also passed laws that prevent genetic discrimination in the provision of health insurance, and represent the primary source of protection. In addition, individuals applying for health insurance are not required to report whether relatives have undergone genetic testing for cancer risk, only whether those relatives have actually been diagnosed with cancer. This information should be conveyed to patients as part of their genetic counseling.

BRCA Genetic Testing

Since genetic testing of the *BRCA* genes first became clinically available in 1996, the published literature on appropriate medical management for patients who test positive has evolved dramatically. Similarly, the approach to offering genetic testing has also evolved. Professional society guidelines outlining when to offer a patient genetic testing for the *BRCA1* and *BRCA2* genes vary among organizations. The American Society of Clinical Oncology (ASCO) position statement on genetic susceptibility testing for cancer was introduced in 1996. It suggested that women with at least a 10% chance of finding a mutation in a breast cancer susceptibility gene were at a high enough risk for genetic testing for inherited breast cancer [143]. These guidelines were updated in 2003, no longer utilizing this 10% cutoff, suggesting that the clinical judgment of a healthcare provider experienced in cancer genetics should be the primary impetus for the appropriateness of genetic testing [130]. Currently, ASCO recommends that genetic testing be offered when (1) the individual has personal or family history features suggestive of a genetic susceptibility condition, (2) the genetic test can be adequately interpreted, (3) the test results will aid in diagnosis or influence the medical management of the patient or family members at hereditary risk of cancer. This is consistent with the guidelines of other professional organizations, most of which provide criteria for outlining which patients should be offered further education and counseling, so that they are able to make informed decisions about genetic testing.

It is more informative for testing of the *BRCA* genes to begin with the patient who is most likely to test positive, typically an individual who had breast cancer at a young age or ovarian cancer. This person should undergo full sequence analysis of both *BRCA1* and *BRCA2* genes and analysis of common large rearrangements in *BRCA1* (e.g. Myriad Genetic Laboratories BRACAanalysis®). If the individual who is being tested is of Ashkenazi Jewish ancestry, the initial analysis should include testing of three founder mutations, 185delAG and 5382insC in *BRCA1*, and 6174delT in *BRCA2*. This approach will be less expensive than comprehensive sequencing (one tenth of the cost), which will be offered if no founding mutation is identified. If a mutation is identified, relatives are usually only tested for that family-specific mutation. Exceptions to this strategy include individuals who present with a significant family history of breast and/or ovarian cancer on both sides of the family. For these individuals, the potential of a different mutation on the opposite side of the family should be addressed, either by offering comprehensive analysis of *BRCA* genes to the individual or the most appropriate affected relative from the opposite side of the family.

Positive Test Result

A positive test is one that discloses the presence of a *BRCA* mutation, which prevents translation of the full-sized protein or is known to interfere in other ways with protein function. Clinically, it means that the individual is at increased risk for breast, ovarian, and other cancers. If the diagnosis of breast or ovarian cancer has already been concluded, then a positive result indicates an increased risk for a possible second primary cancer.

Negative Test Result

A negative test result is interpreted according to an individual's personal and family history, especially with regard to whether a mutation has been previously identified in the family. If a specific mutation has been previously identified in a patient's relative, the patient is tested for that specific mutation. If the mutation is not present, the patient can be reassured that her risk of breast or ovarian cancer is no greater than that of the general population, assuming that there is no history on the other side of the family that might be suggestive of a hereditary cancer syndrome and that there are no other risk factors. In the absence of a previously identified mutation in the family, a negative test result in an affected individual means that the current technology did not find a mutation in *BRCA1* or *BRCA2*. The cause of the pattern of cancer in the patient and the family is still undetermined, and the risk assessment must be based on the clinical history. However, it remains possible that there is an unusual abnormality in one of these genes that has yet to be identified through current technologies. Indeed, it is estimated that clinical testing may not identify up to 15% of mutations within the known susceptibility genes [144].

More recently, Walsh et al. reported that among patients with breast cancer who had significantly family histories of cancer and tested negative for *BRCA1* and *BRCA2*, approximately 12% carried a large genomic deletion or duplication in one of these genes [25]. In this setting, research opportunities should be recommended to families with a significant history of breast and ovarian cancer in which no mutation was identified by commercial testing. It is also possible that the familial cancer is indeed due to an identifiable *BRCA* mutation, but that the individual who tested had sporadic cancer, a situation known as a "phenocopy." This is especially possible if the individual tested developed breast cancer close to the age of onset of the general population (over age 60) rather than before age 50, or if the patient was diagnosed with a cancer than breast or ovarian. In this case, it is recommended that other family members may consider genetic testing. Overall, the false-negative rate for *BRCA* mutational testing is ~5%. It should be noted that there are other possible genes that may be important for the development of genetically based cancer. Mutations within these genes will not be identified with currently available tests that have focused upon the BRCA1 and BRCA2 genes. Although the *BRCA* genes are responsible for the majority of genetically based breast and ovarian cancer, other genes for breast and ovarian cancer susceptibility remain the subject of research. If other specific cancers or clinical findings are present in the patient or family, consideration of various other hereditary cancer syndromes may be warranted.

Indeterminate Test Result

Some test results, especially where a single-base pair change (missense mutation) is identified, may be difficult to interpret. This is because single-base pair changes do not always result in a non-functional gene product. Thus, missense mutations not located within critical functional domains, or those that make only minimal changes in the surrounding protein structure, may not be associated with a clinical disease state, and thus are reported as an indeterminate result. Past studies have shown that many genetic variants in the *BRCA1* and *BRCA2* genes have been reclassified as harmless polymorphisms, with a small number of uncertain variants only later found to be clinically deleterious. Some variants are classified at the outset as "favor polymorphisms" or "suspected deleterious," such that based on the position and type of alteration within the DNA, certain assumptions about the effect upon the protein structure can be made. In communicating indeterminate results with patients, care must be taken to relay the uncertain cancer risk associated with this type of result and emphasize that ongoing research might clarify the meaning of such results. In the case of a "favor polymorphism," the medical management should be based on the strength of the personal and family history of cancer, similar to the approach for a negative mutation in the absence of a known mutation in other relatives. To the contrary, a "suspected deleterious" result may warrant a more aggressive medical management similar to those found to have a mutation, keeping in mind the personal and family history of cancer.

Screening and Risk Management

Effective strategies for the prevention of breast cancer in *BRCA1* and *BRCA2* carriers include: (1) intensive surveillance via screening studies for breast and ovarian cancer, (2) prophylactic surgery (bilateral mastectomy with or without bilateral oophorectomy), and (3) chemoprevention. However, women who are considering interventions to reduce the risk of breast cancer must balance the demonstrated benefits with the potential morbidities of the interventions, since surgical risk reduction strategies may have psychosocial consequences, and chemoprevention, such as tamoxifen and raloxifene, have been associated other potential adverse effects.

Currently, there is no definitive evidence for the true efficacy of screening mammography with regard to the early detection of breast cancer among *BRCA1* and *BRCA2* carriers. Most current screening guidelines are based upon retrospective analyses and large databases rather than prospective data (Table 4.7). Furthermore, the effectiveness of breast self-examination has not been formally evaluated in women with a hereditary risk for breast cancer. In small studies of women with a hereditary risk, the proportion of cancers that were identified solely by clinical screening was 0–4% [145–148]. Similar results have been obtained when breast self-examination is applied to women with an average risk of breast cancer, with no definitive evidence for a reduction in breast-cancer mortality [149].

Mammography-based screening programs that are applied to women with a familial risk of developing breast cancer have not been shown to have an impact on overall survival. The sensitivity of mammography for detecting breast cancer in mutation carriers appears to be lower than in other high-risk groups [145, 147, 150, 151]. The reduced sensitivity of mammography among *BRCA* carriers could possibly be explained by the fact that screening occurs at a younger age compared to the general population. It is well known that this younger patient population has

Table 4.7 Screening and risk reduction recommendations for BRCA mutation carriers

	Recommendation	Frequency
Breast cancer		
Screening	Mammography	Yearly, beginning at age 25
	Breast clinical examination	Every 6 months, beginning at age 25
	Breast self-examination	Monthly, beginning at age 18
	MRI	Yearly, beginning at age 30
Chemoprevention	Tamoxifen/raloxifene	Consider at age 35 and after completion of childbearing
Surgery	Bilateral mastectomy	Consider as an option to screening and tamoxifen
Ovarian cancer		
Screening	Transvaginal ultrasound	Every 6 months, beginning at age 35
	Serum CA 125	Every 6 months, beginning at age 35
Chemoprevention	Oral contraceptives	Consider during childbearing years
Surgery	Bilateral salpingo-oophorectomy	Consider at age 35 and after completion of childbearing

a higher density of breast tissue and in general has a more rapid and aggressive growth of tumors [152]. The development of interval mammographic cancers (those presenting as a palpable mass after normal screening mammography) also tends to be more common in patients with hereditary susceptibility [153]. Microarray analyses of *BRCA1*-associated cancers show a "basal-like" phenotype, which also has been associated with interval mammographic presentations [154].

Despite these limitations in *BRCA* carriers, present screening recommendations for *BRCA* mutation carriers who do not undergo prophylactic mastectomy include clinical breast exam every 3–6 months and mammography every 12 months, beginning between the ages of 25 and 30 years. The risk of developing breast cancer increases significantly after the age of 30. The role of digital mammography has not been fully explored in *BRCA* carriers. The recent Digital Mammographic Imaging Screening Trial (DMIST) reported that this screening modality is more accurate among patients who are younger and with denser breast tissue [155]. This finding may translate into a potential role of digital mammography in screening women who are *BRCA* mutation carriers. Finally, recent studies have raised the issue of potential risks associated with screening recommendations at such an early age [156]. In the IBCCS collaborator's group, any reported exposure to chest X-rays was associated with an increased risk of breast cancer among *BRCA* mutation carriers [157]. Given the central role of *BRCA1* and *BRCA2* in the repair of DNA double-strand breaks, there may be a potential increased risk due to the relatively modest increased exposure to radiation from an increased frequency and duration of mammography. Prospective studies of mutation carriers with detailed mammographic exposure history will be needed to clarify this potential risk associated with mammography exposure at a younger age in *BRCA* carriers.

In the last few years, several prospective and retrospective studies have addressed the role of contrast-enhanced magnetic resonance imaging (MRI) in asymptomatic women at high risk of breast cancer and in women with a hereditary risk for breast cancer [146, 148, 150, 158–164]. These studies suggest that MRI plays an important role in the periodical screening of high-risk women. In a recent review of five prospective studies that assessed the role of screening modalities among women with hereditary predisposition,[165] the pooled sensitivity was 16% for clinical breast examination, 40% for mammography, 43% for ultrasound, and 81% for MRI. The proportion of breast cancers detected only with MRI in prospective studies ranged between 32 and 55%, with a mean of 47%. These studies suggest that at least one-third of all cancers in high-risk populations are deemed occult on clinical breast examination, mammography, and ultrasound but detectable with MRI evaluation. These studies also reveal that interval cancers were found in less than 10% of the patients when MRI was performed, compared to 29% when mammography was utilized.

On the other hand, the proportion of breast cancers that are not detected by MRI, but only by mammography was 12%. It appears that MRI is less sensitive than mammography for detecting ductal carcinoma in situ (DCIS) [146, 148, 164]. In recent years, however, it has become evident that the diagnosis of DCIS is feasible with MRI, although it requires diagnostic criteria that are different from those that are used to diagnose invasive cancer [166]. A recent prospective observational study demonstrated that with the use of a specific diagnostic criteria for DCIS, MRI was more sensitive (98%) in identifying high-grade DCIS compared to mammography (52%) [167]. Therefore, MRI imaging should be considered as a complement to mammography, and be part of the multimodality screening process in high-risk populations [168, 169].

MRI has a lower specificity compared to mammography, which could lead to a higher rate of breast biopsies and additional examinations [146, 161]. In several prospective studies, specificities ranged from 81 to 97% and the positive predictive value ranged between 46 and 63%, with a mean of 53% [165]. The positive predictive value of MRI could be higher in women with hereditary breast cancer susceptibility, and is likely to be most cost-effective for *BRCA1* carriers and for a subgroup of *BRCA2* carriers with dense breast tissue [161, 170]. There are no randomized trials examining the role of breast MRI in mutation carriers and therefore its overall impact on patient outcomes is not known [171]. Despite these concerns, MRI should be discussed as part of a screening strategy, possibly added on as a yearly screening tool in high-risk women and those with *BRCA1* and *BRCA2* gene mutations or carriers. The 2007 guidelines from the American Cancer Society recommend MRI in addition to mammography for women with a lifetime risk of breast cancer greater than approximately 20–25% (*BRCA* mutation carriers), including those with a strong family history of breast or ovarian cancer [111]. Similar guidelines have been recommended by the National Comprehensive Cancer Network (NCCN). The role of ultrasonography in screening *BRCA* mutation carriers has not been well studied, but it has been suggested that ultrasonography may add benefit beyond mammography alone in women with a hereditary risk. It has not been shown to provide any survival benefit in women undergoing screening with MRI [168].

Regarding the risk of ovarian cancer among *BRCA* mutation carriers, it has been recommended that twice yearly transvaginal ultrasound be performed along with serum CA-125 measurements beginning at age 35 for those that have opted to defer prophylactic bilateral oophorectomy [133]. However, these recommendations have not been shown to downstage or improve survival in those patients with ovarian cancer and a *BRCA* mutation [172, 173]. These findings have prompted many clinicians to strongly advocate for bilateral prophylactic oophorectomy at the completion of childbearing rather than intensified screening for ovarian cancer.

Prophylactic Bilateral Mastectomy

In women with *BRCA* mutations, the risk of breast cancer may be reduced with bilateral prophylactic mastectomy and oophorectomy, while risk reduction for ovarian cancer is limited to bilateral oophorectomy (Fig. 4.4). Despite the invasive nature of the intervention, prophylactic mastectomy is the most effective strategy available to absolutely decrease the risk of breast cancer in *BRCA* mutation carriers. In a landmark article by Hartmann et al. they showed a 90% risk reduction in the development of breast cancer in those high-risk patients who underwent bilateral prophylactic mastectomies [174]. Other groups have shown similar efficacy to this procedure associated with this procedure has been demonstrated by several groups [175–177]. The risk reduction may be further reduced up to 95% if women who undergo prior or concurrent bilateral oophorectomy [177].

In one of the first retrospective studies published on this topic, prophylactic mastectomy was performed on women based on family history alone, and women were stratified to moderate and high risk based upon specific methodological outcomes. In 214 high risk women, over a median follow-up period of 14 years, breast cancer was diagnosed in 1.4% of patients [174]. In a follow-up study by the same authors, 26 women from the initial high risk group were identified to be *BRCA1* or *BRCA2* carriers. None of these *BRCA* mutation carriers developed breast cancer during the follow-up period. For only two of the three patients who developed breast cancer, *BRCA1/2* screening was available. In this select group, prophylactic mastectomy yielded an estimated overall breast cancer risk reduction of 89.5–100%, considering the patient with unknown screening as both mutation carrier and a noncarrier [175]. A more recent prospective study among *BRCA* mutation carriers showed that breast cancer was diagnosed in 2% of patients who had prophylactic mastectomy compared to 49% in the control group, thus reducing the risk of breast cancer by approximately 90–95% [177].

However, a simple mastectomy does not remove 100% of the breast tissue, with an average of 3–5% remaining within the superior and inferior skin flaps. Thus, this remaining tissue is still at risk for the future development of breast cancer as the germline mutations are present in any remaining breast tissue. The absolute risk after bilateral prophylactic mastectomy has not been clearly defined. Studies are currently underway to determine the impact of prophylactic mastectomy on overall and cancer-specific survival. Among women with unilateral breast cancer, at least one study suggests that prophylactic contralateral mastectomy improves both cancer-specific and "all-cause" survival [178]. Prophylactic mastectomy is recommended in the form of simple mastectomy, since the risk of leaving breast tissue

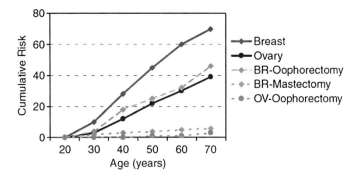

Fig. 4.4 Cancer risk reduction with prophylactic surgery (adapted with permission from Domchek SM, Weber BL. Clinical management of *BRCA1* and *BRCA2* carriers. Oncogene 2006;25:5825–5831)

behind is lower compared to subcutaneous mastectomy [177, 179–181]. However, many women do not find this strategy acceptable for cosmetic reasons. Therefore, procedures that involve a skin-sparing mastectomy with or without preservation of the nipple–areolar complex with immediate reconstruction are now more commonly being offered in the management of breast cancer risk reduction among *BRCA* mutation carriers. This type of prophylactic mastectomy appears to provide superior cosmetic results, and appears to be a reasonable compromise in breast cancer risk reduction [181]. However, oncological failures can occur in the nipple–areolar complex as a result of residual at-risk tissue in the breast. Prospective comparative studies with long-term follow-up are needed to precisely establish the risks of cancer after simple mastectomy, subcutaneous, and skin-sparing mastectomy with preservation of the nipple–areolar complex.

Prophylactic Bilateral Oophorectomy

Oophorectomy is the single most important intervention available to *BRCA* mutation carriers to reduce the risk of ovarian cancer, as there is really no effective ovarian cancer screening tools currently available. Although this surgery has not been formally evaluated in randomized trials, retrospective and prospective studies indicate a reduction in the risk of *BRCA*-associated gynecologic cancers of 80–96% with a risk reduction in the development of breast cancer of approximately 50%, most likely through the induction of premature menopause [182–185]. In fact, the significant effect of bilateral oophorectomy on reducing the breast cancer risk may partially explain the variability in penetrance estimates for breast cancer across studies. The reduction in breast cancer risk appears greatest when oophorectomy is performed before the age of 40 and its protective effect appears evident at least 15 years following surgery [185]. This procedure is also associated with reduced overall and cancer-specific survival [186].

It is recommended that *BRCA* mutation carriers undergo prophylactic oophorectomy after the age of 35 or once childbearing is completed. Removal of both fallopian tubes should also be performed due to the potential risk of developing fallopian tube carcinoma. Similar to prophylactic mastectomy, prophylactic oophorectomy does not completely eliminate risk. Primary peritoneal cancers have been reported in women with *BRCA* mutations following prophylactic oophorectomy with an estimated frequency of 2–4%, occurring more frequently in *BRCA1* compared to *BRCA2* carriers [184, 187]. Despite the multiple benefits associated with bilateral oophorectomy, some women delay or refuse oophorectomy owing to fear of symptoms related to surgical menopause. Furthermore, there is a theoretical concern that short-term low estrogen replacement may reduce the protective effect against breast cancer. Recent studies have reported that short-term hormone replacement therapy after prophylactic oophorectomy in premenopausal women with no history of breast cancer does not impact breast cancer risk [188]. Further studies are underway to determine whether timing, type, or duration of hormonal replacement therapy have significant effects upon breast cancer reduction in *BRCA* mutation carriers.

Chemoprevention

Chemoprevention strategies among women at high risk for breast cancer involve the use of selective estrogen receptor modulators (tamoxifen and raloxifene), while oral contraceptives have been used for chemoprevention of ovarian cancer. However, there is only limited data available regarding specific chemoprevention strategies for *BRCA* mutation carriers. Tamoxifen was the first drug shown to reduce the incidence of breast cancer in women at high risk for this disease. The National Surgical Adjuvant Breast and Bowel Project (NSABP) P-1 trial (Breast Cancer Prevention Trial) randomly assigned more than 13,000 women with a 5-year risk of breast cancer of 1.66% or more to tamoxifen or placebo based on the Gail model [189]. After a mean follow-up of 4 years, tamoxifen was found to reduce the incidence of breast cancer by 49%. In women aged 49 years or younger, the decreased risk occurred in 44% of patients who were randomized to tamoxifen, with a risk reduction in non-invasive breast cancer of 50%. Overall, tamoxifen resulted in a 50% risk reduction for breast cancer in women who had a strong family history of breast cancer.

Serious side effects related to tamoxifen include venous thromboembolism, endometrial cancer, and development of cataracts. A subsequent subgroup analysis of the NSABP-P1 trial suggested a non-significant protective effect of tamoxifen for *BRCA2* carriers, but not among *BRCA1* carriers [190]. It was concluded that a true benefit of tamoxifen in *BRCA* carriers cannot be excluded given the small number of mutation carriers in the study population. On the other hand, tamoxifen has been shown in case–control and prospective studies to decrease the risk of contralateral breast cancer by almost 50% among *BRCA* carriers who have been diagnosed with breast cancer [190–194]. This effect was seen in both pre- and postmenopausal women.

It has been suggested that there may be a selective benefit of tamoxifen in *BRCA2* carriers compared to *BRCA1* carriers. The NSABP-P1 trial demonstrated that tamoxifen reduced the occurrence of estrogen receptor-positive tumors by 69%, but no difference in the occurrence of estrogen receptor-negative tumors was seen. Between 17 and 24% of breast tumors among *BRCA1* carriers are estrogen receptor-positive, compared to 76–78% of *BRCA2* associated tumors. However, the benefit of adjuvant tamoxifen therapy has been observed among *BRCA1* mutation carriers with breast cancer, irrespective of estrogen receptor status [191, 195]. Therefore, it is not yet clear whether tamoxifen exerts differential effects in *BRCA1* compared to *BRCA2* mutation carriers. Thus, until further information is available, mutation carriers may be offered tamoxifen as a chemoprevention option for breast cancer risk reduction.

In the subsequent NSABP study of tamoxifen and raloxifene (STAR) P-2 trial, raloxifene was shown to be as effective as tamoxifen in reducing the risk of invasive breast cancer. However, there was a non-statistically significant higher risk of non-invasive breast cancer (ductal or lobular carcinoma in situ) in postmenopausal women at high risk [196]. Raloxifene was associated with a lower risk of endometrial cancer and venous thromboembolism, but the application of raloxifene in premenopausal women is not recommended due to the increased incidence of ovarian cysts [197]. Finally, the effect of raloxifene in *BRCA* mutation carriers has not been studied.

The use of oral contraceptives appears to decrease the risk of ovarian cancer by up to 60% in *BRCA1* and *BRCA2* carriers in several case–control studies, although one report did not find this effect [198–201]. However, other studies have suggested that oral contraceptives may increase the risk of breast cancer in mutation carriers [202–204]. Therefore, it is possible that oral contraceptives have a dual impact upon cancer risk in *BRCA* carriers, providing a degree of protection for ovarian cancer, but increasing the risk of breast cancer. Given the high mortality associated with ovarian cancer compared with breast cancer, a reasonable risk reduction strategy may be the use of oral contraceptives before childbearing and subsequently followed by bilateral prophylactic oophorectomy once childbearing has been completed.

Clinical Characteristics and Management of *BRCA1* and *BRCA2* Associated Breast Cancer

Many studies have tried to identify characteristics that are unique in respect to hereditary breast cancer syndromes compared to sporadic cases. The general notion is that these subsets of breast cancer manifest with their own unique behavior and natural history (Table 4.8). It is well known that women with mutations of either *BRCA1* or *BRCA2* have an increased risk of developing other cancers, such as breast, ovarian, fallopian, and peritoneal cancers.

Table 4.8 Characteristics of BRCA1- and BRCA2-associated breast cancers

Characteristic	BRCA1	BRCA2
Incidence/penetrance	45% of hereditary breast cancer, highly penetrant, conferring a breast cancer risk of about 57% by age 70 (95% CI, 47–66%)	35% of hereditary breast cancer, highly penetrant, conferring a breast cancer risk of about 49% by age 70 (95% CI, 40–57%)
Tumor spectrum	Female breast cancer, ovarian cancer, possibly colon, and prostate	Female breast cancer, ovarian cancer, male breast cancer, colon cancer, prostate cancer, pancreatic cancer, gallbladder, bile duct, and stomach cancer, malignant melanoma
Genotype–phenotype	The risks for breast and ovarian cancer are related to the position of the mutation, with truncating mutations in the first two-thirds of the coding region being associated with a higher ovarian cancer risk, relative to breast cancer risk, than mutations in the last third	Truncating mutations indentified in the families with the highest risk of ovarian cancer relative to breast cancer are clustered in a region of approximately 3.3 kb in exon 11 "ovarian cancer cluster region"
Somatic mutations	Infrequent in primary breast and ovarian carcinomas	Infrequent in primary breast and ovarian carcinomas
Primary breast cancer	Early age of onset, high prevalence of bilateral cancer (up to 65%), "triple negative phenotype" (ER/PR/HER2 negative), higher proliferative activity, poor histological differentiation, lower frequency of nodal metastases, fewer recurrences	Early age of onset, high prevalence of bilateral cancer (up to 50%), lower proliferative activity, well-differentiated histological characteristics

BRCA1

In general, mutations within the human germline have a high level of penetrance, strongly associated with breast, ovarian, fallopian, peritoneal, colon, and prostate cancers. These cancers are associated with an early age of onset (approximately 20% develop breast cancer before age 40, and one-half by the age of 50), increased risk of bilateral breast cancer (up to 65%), higher proliferation activity, poorly differentiated, estrogen receptor negativity, and HER2/neu negativity [205–207]. Poor differentiation, high tumor grade with aneuploidy, negative hormone receptors, and a mutation of the p53 gene have been identified as negative prognostic variables. There appears to be a lower frequency of nodal metastases and fewer local recurrences after resection of the primary cancer. A recent study found that axillary nodal status did not significantly correlate with tumor size of the primary lesion in *BRCA1* carriers, a finding that is significant in women with sporadic breast cancer or *BRCA2* mutations [208, 209].

There is less information regarding if women are at increased risk of endometrial cancer. A recent study evaluated 857 women with deleterious mutations of *BRCA1* and *BRCA2* for the incidence of endometrial cancer. Over a period of 3.3 years, six women were diagnosed with endometrial cancer, as compared to an expected 1.13 cancers. It should be noted that four of these women had previously received adjuvant tamoxifen therapy for treatment of their breast cancers. The authors concluded that women with *BRCA* mutations who had previously received tamoxifen may be considered for prophylactic hysterectomy [210].

BRCA2

A mutation within the BRCA2 gene can be associated with breast, ovarian, pancreatic, gallbladder cancer, cholangiocarcinoma, gastric cancer, and melanoma. It also confers an increased prevalence of male breast cancer. Clinical characteristics are similar to *BRCA1* such as an early age of onset and an increased risk of bilateral breast cancer. However, in contradistinction to *BRCA1*, *BRCA2* tumors generally have a lower proliferative activity and tend to well-differentiated on pathologic analysis.

Histopathology

A large amount of research has recently emerged demonstrating that primary breast cancers from patients with germline *BRCA1* and *BRCA2* genetic mutations are morphologically and genetically different from each other. Invasive ductal carcinoma is the most common histological subtype in hereditary breast cancer as well as in sporadic cancers. In *BRCA1*, there is a higher incidence of medullary carcinoma of 11%, compared to a 2% rate for the *BRCA2* gene and 1% for sporadic cancers [211]. Both medullary and atypical medullary carcinomas have been found to lead to a favorable prognosis. *BRCA2* tumors do not seem to have a clear association with a specific histologic subtype of breast cancer as compared to *BRCA1*. Some studies have demonstrated that invasive lobular, pleomorphic lobular, tubular, and cribiform types arise more frequently than sporadic tumors [212–214]. However, other series have reported no statistical difference in histologic subtypes in *BRCA2* as compared to sporadic cancers [70, 215]. Higher percentages of premalignant lesions such as atypical lobular and ductal hyperplasia, lobular, and ductal carcinoma in situ have been found in specimens from women with hereditary *BRCA1/2* mutations who previously underwent bilateral prophylactic mastectomy [216, 217].

It appears that mutations within the *BRCA1* gene are associated with a higher tumor grade, mitotic rate, nuclear polymorphism, less tubule formation, lower p27 (Kip1) protein levels, and cyclin E expression as compared to *BRCA2* [218, 219]. Greater than 70% of *BRCA1* tumors are grade 3, as compared to 35% of sporadic cancers [211, 212, 220–223]. Glomeruloid microvascular proliferation, a marker of tumor vascularity, is significantly more likely to be present in *BRCA1* tumors, as well as MYC amplification [224–226]. *BRCA1* carriers had less ductal carcinoma in situ around the invasive lesion compared to control lesions, with lobular carcinoma in situ less common in familial cancers.

BRCA1 tumors are more likely to be estrogen receptor (ER), progesterone receptor (PR), and HER2/neu negative (triple negative phenotype) and harbor mutations in TP53 than matched sporadic cancers [215, 227]. Between 63 and 90% of *BRCA1* tumors are ER negative, and PR is more frequently negative when compared to *BRCA2* and sporadic tumors [220, 227–235]. In comparison, *BRCA2* tumors are ER positive in 60–90% of cases and PR positive in 40–80% which is similar to sporadic tumors [212, 223, 227–229, 233, 234]. HER2/neu expression in *BRCA1* and *BRCA2* is generally very low, at less than 3% of all cases examined [227, 228, 236]. Some authors have hypothesized that HER2/neu over-expression may not be associated with *BRCA* mutations due to a possible co-deletion of *BRCA1* and HER2/neu loci. Other possibilities point toward changes in chromatin conformation or possibly that *BRCA* tumors evolved through genetic pathways whereby gains of HER2/neu function did not confer a survival advantage to neoplastic cells [237–239].

When comparing *BRCA2* cancers with sporadic cancers, tumors are of higher overall grade with less tubule formation, with no significant difference noted in the number of mitoses, pleomorphism, steroid receptor expression, or TP53 mutation [239]. Numerous genes have been examined in an attempt to differentiate *BRCA1*, *BRCA2*, and sporadic tumor from each other (Table 4.9). *BRCA2* tumors are more likely to have expression of cyclin D1 compared to *BRCA1* and sporadic tumors [240, 241]. In 2005, tissues collected from the International Breast Cancer Linkage Consortium with *BRCA1* and *BRCA2* mutations were analyzed for basal

Table 4.9 Immunophenotype of *BRCA1*, *BRCA2*, and sporadic breast cancer

Antibodies	BRCA1	BRCA2	Sporadic
ER, PR	-	+	+
BCL-2, BAX	-	+	+
Cyclin D1	-	+	+
p16, p27, p21	-	+	+
RAD50	-	+	+
RAD51 (cytoplasm)	-	+	-
HER2	-	-	+
CHEK2	+	+	-
RAD51 (nucleus)	+	-	+
P53, Ki-67	+	-	-
Cyclins (E, A, B1)	+	-	-
Skp2	+	-	-
CK 5/6, 14, 17	+	-	-
EGFR, p-cadherin	+	-	-

Source: Adapted with permission from Honrado E, Osorio A, Palacios J and Benitez J. Pathology and gene expression of hereditary breast tumors associated with *BRCA1*, *BRCA2* and CHEK2 gene mutations. Oncogene 2006; 25:5837–5845

markers to help identify predictive histological characteristics of these mutations. The authors found five relevant markers, CK5/6, CK14, CK17, osteonectin, and epidermal growth factor receptor (EGFR) to be statistically significant when comparing *BRCA1* to sporadic tumors as controls. In multivariate analysis, CK5/6, CK14, and ER were predictors of *BRCA1* carrier status. *BRCA2* tumors did not differ in staining as compared to controls [242]. An additional set of genetic markers have recently been found to be expressed in *BRCA1* tumors which are not considered basal markers, these include cyclin E, p53, Skp2, and negativity for p27 [235, 242–244].

Surgical Treatment Options

In the past decade, numerous studies have explored the role of breast conserving therapy compared to mastectomy when treating patients with hereditary breast cancer. There has been some controversy in the literature regarding the use of breast conserving therapy in *BRCA* carriers, due to the suggested higher risk of in-breast tumor recurrence [192, 245–249]. There is a defined risk of second primary breast cancers in association with *BRCA1* and *BRCA2* mutations, both in the ipsilateral and contralateral breast. Recent data on 160 *BRCA1* and *BRCA2* carriers who underwent breast conserving treatment compared to 445 matched controls revealed no statistically significant difference in ipsilateral breast cancer recurrence between the two groups [192]. The 10- and 15-year estimates for ipsilateral recurrence were 12 and 24% in the *BRCA* carriers and 9 and 17% in the controls, with a median follow-up of 7.9 years. The incidence of ipsilateral breast cancers in carriers who had undergone bilateral oophorectomy was not significantly different compared to the control group. However, contralateral breast cancers were significantly greater in *BRCA* carriers versus controls. Ten- and 15-year estimates of contralateral breast cancer were 26 and 39% for carriers compared to 3 and 7% for controls. In addition, tamoxifen use significantly reduced the risk of contralateral breast cancer in *BRCA* carriers.

Another study reviewed breast conserving therapy in 87 patients with *BRCA* mutations [248]. They found 5- and 10-year estimates for metachronous ipsilateral breast cancer to be 11.2 and 13.6%, respectively, with rates for metachronous contralateral breast cancer of 11.9 and 37.6%. This rate for ipsilateral breast cancer is similar to those reported in women with sporadic breast cancers. Another group published their experience with breast conserving therapy in 87 patients with hereditary breast cancer, 26 of which were known *BRCA1* or *BRCA2* carriers [249]. These patients were compared to 174 patients with sporadic tumors treated in the same period with breast conserving therapy. At a median follow-up of 6.1 years, the observed ipsilateral breast tumor recurrence rate was 21.8% in the hereditary groups and 12.1% in the sporadic group. The estimated rate of ipsilateral breast tumor recurrence was found to be significantly higher in the hereditary breast cancer group at both 5 and 10 years.

Role of Prophylactic Contralateral Mastectomy

Both retrospective and prospective analyses have shown an approximately 90% or greater decrease in the risk of developing breast cancer in *BRCA1* and *BRCA2* carriers after undergoing bilateral prophylactic mastectomy [174, 176, 177]. A recent retrospective study evaluated the role of contralateral prophylactic mastectomy in patients diagnosed with invasive breast cancer [178]. They compared 1,072 women who underwent contralateral prophylactic mastectomy to a matched group of 317 women who did not undergo contralateral prophylactic mastectomy. At a median follow-up of 5.7 years, contralateral breast cancer developed in 0.5% of women with contralateral prophylactic mastectomy, and 8.1% died of breast cancer. In contrast, contralateral breast cancer developed in 2.7% of women without contralateral prophylactic mastectomy, and 11.7% died of breast cancer. The authors concluded that contralateral prophylactic mastectomy decreased the incidence of contralateral breast cancer, subsequently resulting in a decrease in overall breast cancer mortality.

Adjuvant Therapy

The standard utility for the use of systemic adjuvant therapy for breast cancer in *BRCA* mutation carriers remains similar to that of sporadic cancers, although this notion is changing. Currently, chemotherapeutic regimens are based more on histopathologic characteristics of the primary tumor rather than underlying genetic mutations. There has never been a prospective, randomized controlled trial addressing the role of chemotherapy in *BRCA* carriers. Nonetheless, there have been some smaller studies suggesting that platinum-based therapies may be more effective than taxanes in *BRCA* carriers, with others questioning the role of anthracyclines in this setting. There has been interest in the hypothesis that the functional effects as a result of loss in *BRCA1* and *BRCA2* expression may influence the response to specific cancer drugs [56, 250, 251]. Further clinical trials will be needed to truly answer this important question, with some evidence suggesting that *BRCA1* may act as modulator of chemotherapy-induced apoptosis [250]. Others hypothesize that the loss of function of *BRCA1* is associated with sensitivity to DNA-damaging chemotherapy and possibly associated with taxane resistance [251]. A European phase 2 randomized trial comparing carboplatin and docetaxel in *BRCA*-associated metastatic breast cancer patients is currently accruing patients in order to address these hypotheses in the clinical setting.

A small study looking at neoadjuvant chemotherapy in breast cancer patients with either *BRCA1/2* mutations found an improved clinical response compared to non-carriers, with a higher percentage of complete responders in *BRCA* carriers, independent of tumor stage [252]. After three or four cycles of neoadjuvant chemotherapy, a complete response was recorded in 10/11 *BRCA1/2* carriers (93%) compared with 8/27 non-carriers (30%). Others have shown that both basal tumors (*BRCA1*-like) and HER2/neu positive cancers were the only breast cancers to have a greater responses to neoadjuvant chemotherapy [253].

It has also been shown that 67% of *BRCA1*-positive breast cancers express the epidermal growth factor receptor (EGFR), as compared to 21% of sporadic cases [242]. This increased expression may lead to a potential benefit with the use of targeted therapies against the EGFR receptor, such as cetuximab or small molecule tyrosine kinase inhibitors gefitinib or erlotinib. A newer strategy utilizing targeted therapy in *BRCA* tumors is the use of Poly (ADP-ribose) polymerase (PARP) inhibitors [254–257]. The absence of PARP leads to spontaneous single-strand DNA breaks which progress to double-strand breaks with resultant repair. The summary effect once both the *BRCA* genes and PARP pathways are inhibited leads to chromosomal instability, cell cycle arrest, and subsequent apoptosis. PARP inhibitors are now being investigated in clinical trials in combination with various cytotoxic agents [258, 259].

The first evidence of the clinical importance of HER2/neu over-expression in breast cancer came from a report of HER2/neu gene amplification in poor prognosis breast cancer [260]. Examination of the extent of HER2/neu activation via phosphorylation can stratify patients into good versus poor prognostic groups. A large phase III study of patients with metastatic breast cancer who were randomized to chemotherapy with or without Herceptin (trastuzumab) showed a doubling of the response rate and a significant prolongation of disease-free progression in those patients who received Herceptin. This led to the United States Food and Drug Administration approval of Herceptin as one of the first targeted therapies for patients with HER2/neu overexpressing breast cancer, either as a first-line agent in combination with paclitaxel or as a second- or third-line single therapy in the metastatic setting. However, due to low HER2/neu expression in most *BRCA* related tumors, the utility of Herceptin is somewhat limited in this subset of patients.

Prognosis

Historically it has been felt that *BRCA1* related breast tumors led to poorer survival outcomes as compared to matched sporadic and *BRCA2* control groups. A single cohort study showed that there is an adverse prognosis associated with patients with *BRCA1*-positive breast cancer that did not receive chemotherapy compared to historical controls [252]. Recently, a Dutch study evaluated 49 patients with proven *BRCA1* mutations and compared clinical outcomes with a matched group of patients with sporadic breast cancer [261]. In this series, *BRCA1*-associated breast cancers had twice as many PR-negative tumors with a four- to fivefold increased incidence of developing contralateral breast cancer. There was no statistically significant difference found in disease-free survival at 5 years in the *BRCA1* group (49%) compared to the sporadic group (51%), with an overall 5-year survival rate of 63 and 69% respectively. A population based study from Israel was designed to determine the influence of *BRCA1* and *BRCA2* mutations on prognosis in breast cancer [262]. The adjusted hazard ratios for death from breast cancer were not statistically significant when comparing mutation carriers to sporadic cases. For Non-*BRCA* hereditary breast cancers, it is felt that they have a less aggressive presentation but the prognostic implication of this has not been studied in large series [209].

Other Hereditary Syndromes Associated with Breast Cancer

Li-Fraumeni Syndrome (P53)

The first description of the syndrome was by Li and Fraumeni in 1969 in a retrospective review of more than 600 pediatric patients with sarcoma [263]. This rare autosomal dominant condition is associated with soft tissue sarcomas, early onset breast cancer, childhood leukemia, osteosarcoma, melanoma, colon cancer, pancreatic cancer, adrenocortical carcinoma, and brain cancers, diagnosed before the age of 45 years. In 1990, the Li-Fraumeni syndrome was associated with mutations within the p53 gene, which is demonstrated in approximately half of all known families with this syndrome [264]. Up to 50% of carriers develop some form of cancer by the age of 30, with 90% developing cancer by the age of 70 [265]. The incidence of breast cancer in women with Li-Fraumeni Syndrome with germline p53 mutations who survive childhood cancers is approximately 22–50% by the age of 50, with a lifetime penetrance of 100% [266]. In addition, there is a 25% risk of multiple breast cancers and of other primary tumors [267]. Predictive testing may be considered for at-risk family members when a mutation is identified in an affected proband.

Cowden's Disease (PTEN)

Cowden's disease is a rare autosomal dominant mutation which predisposes patients to both benign and malignant neoplasms including: trichilemmomas, mucocutanous papillomatous papules, macrocephaly, and an increased risk of breast, thyroid, endometrial, and cerebellar tumors. It was first reported by Lloyd and Dennis in 1963, who named the disease after their patient Rachel Cowden [268]. The disease is caused by a germline mutation in the PTEN gene (MMAC1/TEP1), which is a tumor suppressor gene on chromosome 10q23.3 [269–271]. The lifetime risk of breast cancer in women with Cowden's disease is estimated to be as high as 50%, with adenocarcinoma being the most common histologic subtype. There is also an increased incidence of male breast cancer [272–274].

Peutz-Jeghers Syndrome (STK11/LKB1)

Peutz-Jeghers Syndrome is associated with a germline mutation in STK11/LKB1, a serine threonine kinase located on chromosome 19p13.3 [275, 276]. Patients with the syndrome present with hamartomatous polyps throughout the small bowel and pigmented buccal mucosa, lips, fingers, and toes. A recent analysis of the incidence of cancers in 419 patients with the syndrome found the STK11/LKB1 mutation present in 70% of patients [277]. Over 85% these mutations (missense or truncating) were localized to regions of STK11/LKB1 encoding the kinase domain of the expressed protein. A total of 96 malignant tumors were confirmed in the studied population. The most common cancers were of gastrointestinal origin including; gastroesophageal, small bowel, colon, and pancreatic. In women with Peutz-Jeghers syndrome, the incidence of breast cancer was increased with 8 and 31% at 40 and 60 years of age, respectively. The presence of the STK11/LKB1 mutation does not appear to affect the incidence of cancer in patients with Peutz-Jeghers syndrome.

Muir-Torre Syndrome (MSH2/MLH1)

Muir-Torre syndrome is defined by the presence of sebaceous gland and visceral malignancies. It has an autosomal dominant inheritance with high penetrance [71]. In the Muir-Torre syndrome, the most common malignancy is colorectal cancer arising in ~50% of effected patients, with 25% of female carriers developing breast cancer at a median age of 68. This syndrome is most frequently found as a variant of the autosomal dominant disorder hereditary non-polyposis colorectal cancer (HNPCC) syndrome, with tumors demonstrating microsatellite instability and germline mutations in the DNA mismatch repair genes MSH2 and MLH1.

Ataxia Telangiectasia (ATM)

Ataxia telangiectasia is an autosomal recessive disorder associated with cerebellar ataxia, telangiectasia, immunodeficiencies, radiation sensitivity, and predisposition to cancers in general. This is due to homozygous mutations in the ATM gene. Epidemiologic studies of ataxia telangiectasia families suggest that ATM carriers may have an increased risk ratio for the development of breast cancer of approximately 3.3–3.9:1, although this observation is somewhat controversial [278–286].

CHEK2

Recent research suggests that CHEK2 serves as an integral component of the molecular pathways involved with ataxia telangiectasia and has been identified in 5% of patients with non-BRCA hereditary breast cancer, including Li-Fraumeni Syndrome [287]. Germline CHEK2 mutations including the CHEK2 *1100delC mutation are associated with a two- to threefold increase risk of developing breast cancer, and may put patients at increased risk of second primary breast cancers and poorer overall outcomes [239, 287–289].

P450 Gene CYP1A1

The gene CYP1A1 encodes for aryl hydrocarbon hydroxylase, which is the primary enzymatic catalyst for the conversion of estradiol to hydroxylated estrogen [290]. Reduction in estrogen exposure is protective for the development of breast cancer, whereas increased estrogen exposure can increase this risk. Alterations in the activity of aryl hydrocarbon hydroxylase can thus lead to variations in the serum levels of estrogen, affecting the overall risk of developing breast cancer. A particular allelic variant, found in 14% of carriers with breast cancer and 22% of unaffected carriers, reduced the risk of breast cancer by about 40%. Studies addressing the role of this gene and an interaction with BRCA1/2 genes are underway.

Glutathione S-Transferases

The glutathione S-transferases constitute a family of genes that encode enzymes that catalyze the conjunction of reactive chemical intermediates to soluble glutathione conjugates to facilitate clearance. There are four classes of cytosolic glutathione S-transferases, of which at least three are expressed in normal breast tissue [291]. The glutathione S-transferases have a null polymorphism that results in a total lack of enzyme production in 50% of the population. Due to the fact that these enzymes metabolize environmental carcinogens, there has been increased interest in determining whether homozygotes for the null allele have an increased risk of breast cancer [292].

N-Acetyltransferase

Polymorphisms in the N-acetyltransferase genes, specifically NAT2, are associated with an altered rate of metabolism of carcinogens. Wild-type alleles define a rapid acetylator phenotype, whereas homozygosity for any combination of the three variant alleles results in a slow acetylator phenotype. This slow phenotype may lead to altered metabolism of carcinogenic amines. The combination of smoking and slow acetylator status in *BRCA1* mutation carriers has been shown to result in an increased incidence of breast cancer [293]. Altered steroid hormone metabolism may contribute to this increased incidence.

Low-Penetrant Breast Cancer Susceptibility Genes

Low-penetrant susceptibility alleles, or "modifier genes" are defined as polymorphic genes with specific alleles that are associated with an altered risk for disease susceptibility. Although each variant is associated with only a small increase in the risk for breast cancer in any individual, the attributed risk in the general population is likely to be higher than for genes which are rarer with high-penetrant susceptibility. Although many investigators are researching these genes, the role of modifier genes in breast cancer remains unclear [19].

Gene Expression Profilling

Many groups have utilized gene expression profiling of breast cancers to provide unique information regarding the differences between *BRCA1*, *BRCA2*, and sporadic cancers [254, 294–296]. Studying tumors at the genetic level may help to further stratify staging, improve treatment, and elucidate new molecular pathways and to help identify future therapeutic targets. Using microarray, five breast cancer subtypes were identified and validated in both clinically and ethnically diverse patient populations [297–300]. These five subtypes include basal-like (which is associated to *BRCA1* and the "triple negative phenotype"), HER2-overexpressing, luminal A, luminal B, and normal breast-like. These subtypes have been compared to clinical outcomes, with a significantly worse prognosis identified in those patents with basal-like or HER2-overexpressed tumors compared to luminal A tumors [298, 299, 301, 302].

Molecular profiling has been used to stratify breast cancer patients into prognostic groups. Mammaprint (Agendia BV, Amsterdam, the Netherlands) is a diagnostic test which utilizes freshly procured breast cancer samples, comprised of a 70-gene breast cancer signature that is capable of stratifying patients into prognostic groups. This was originally designed by comparing the gene expression patterns in node-negative breast cancer patients who were less than 55 years of age, with T1 or T2 primary tumors who developed metastases within 5 years of diagnosis. They compared this group to a matched group that did not develop metastasis. This gene signature has since been validated with an independent dataset, and is currently being utilized in the MINDACT trial (Microarray In Node negative Disease may Avoid ChemoTherapy) which is actively accruing patients [303–306].

Oncotype Dx® (Genomic Health Inc, Redwood City, CA) is a 21-gene reverse-transcriptase polymerase chain reaction (RT-PCR) assay that utilizes the paraffin-embedded tumor blocks of the primary breast cancer, with 15 cancer-related genes and 6 reference genes. It is commercially available test that is able to predict the recurrence rates of breast cancer patients at 10 years time. It should be noted that this test has only been validated for patients who are node-negative and ER-positive. The assay determines a true recurrence score at 10 years, which stratifies patients into low, intermediate, or a high-risk of recurrence [295, 307]. Currently, this assay is being studied in a clinical trial (Trial Assigning IndividuaLized Options for Treatment - TAILORx), evaluating the role of chemotherapy in node-negative patients. Patients with a high score are given chemotherapy and hormone therapy, while patients in the low-risk group are treated with hormonal therapy only. The study group for the TAILORx trial is comprised of those patients in the intermediate group, which are then randomized to receive hormonal therapy alone or combination chemotherapy plus hormonal therapy [306].

Genomic technology has a fairly high accuracy rate of ~84% to distinguish *BRCA1* tumors from sporadic breast tumors [308]. In addition, it has been shown, using array-based comparative genomics, that *BRCA1* tumors have a higher frequency of copy number alterations as compared to sporadic cancers. They have found frequent losses of 4p, 4q, 5q which were used to correctly classify *BRCA1* from *BRCA2* tumors [309]. Recently, a *BRCA1* genetic signature has been studied which used gene expression profiling to identify patients with a "poor prognosis" signature in breast tumors with node negative disease [303]. Using a set of 100 genes, researchers were able to distinguish *BRCA1* from sporadic ER-negative breast cancers with a 95% accuracy rate.

With the advent of complex molecular diagnostic techniques, such as cDNA microarray, fluorescence in situ hybridization (FISH), comparative genomic hybridization (CGH), and spectral karyotyping (SKY) analysis, it will soon be possible to identify several new genetic abnormalities in patients with breast cancer. This will ultimately facilitate a better understanding of the *BRCA* genes and exactly how they are involved with the development of breast cancer. As new factors and genes are being discovered, we may begin to explain phenomena such as incomplete penetrance, as we observe that not every *BRCA* germline mutation carrier will develop breast or ovarian cancer. This could be explained by molecular pathways that have not yet been elucidated and potentially compensate for the loss of crucial *BRCA* co-factors or signaling pathways that lead to tumorigenesis in *BRCA* mutation carriers.

References

1. Kamangar F, Dores GM, Anderson WF. Patterns of cancer incidence, mortality, and prevalence across five continents: defining priorities to reduce cancer disparities in different geographic regions of the world. J Clin Oncol 2006;24:2137–50.
2. Jemal A, Siegel R, Ward E, Murray T, Xu J, Thun MJ. Cancer statistics, 2007. CA Cancer J Clin 2007;57:43–66.
3. Jemal A, Ward E, Thun MJ. Recent trends in breast cancer incidence rates by age and tumor characteristics among U.S. women. Breast Cancer Res 2007;9:R28.
4. Antoniou AC, Easton DF. Models of genetic susceptibility to breast cancer. Oncogene 2006;25:5898–905.
5. Colditz GA, Willett WC, Hunter DJ, et al. Family history, age, and risk of breast cancer. Prospective data from the Nurses' Health Study. JAMA 1993;270:338–43.
6. Slattery ML, Kerber RA. A comprehensive evaluation of family history and breast cancer risk. The Utah Population Database. JAMA 1993;270:1563–8.
7. Claus EB, Risch NJ, Thompson WD. Age at onset as an indicator of familial risk of breast cancer. Am J Epidemiol 1990;131:961–72.
8. Anderson DE, Badzioch MD. Combined effect of family history and reproductive factors on breast cancer risk. Cancer 1989;63:349–53.
9. Narod SA. Modifiers of risk of hereditary breast and ovarian cancer. Nat Rev Cancer 2002;2:113–23.
10. Kramer JL, Velazquez IA, Chen BE, Rosenberg PS, Struewing JP, Greene MH. Prophylactic oophorectomy reduces breast cancer penetrance during prospective, long-term follow-up of BRCA1 mutation carriers. J Clin Oncol 2005;23:8629–35.

11. Brose MS, Rebbeck TR, Calzone KA, Stopfer JE, Nathanson KL, Weber BL. Cancer risk estimates for BRCA1 mutation carriers identified in a risk evaluation program. J Natl Cancer Inst 2002;94:1365–72.

12. Easton DF, Bishop DT, Ford D, Crockford GP. Genetic linkage analysis in familial breast and ovarian cancer: results from 214 families. The Breast Cancer Linkage Consortium. Am J Hum Genet 1993;52:678–701.

13. Antoniou A, Pharoah PD, Narod S, et al. Average risks of breast and ovarian cancer associated with BRCA1 or BRCA2 mutations detected in case Series unselected for family history: a combined analysis of 22 studies. Am J Hum Genet 2003;72:1117–30.

14. Anglian Breast Cancer Study Group. Prevalence and penetrance of BRCA1 and BRCA2 mutations in a population-based series of breast cancer cases. Br J Cancer 2000;83: 1301–8.

15. Struewing JP, Hartge P, Wacholder S, et al. The risk of cancer associated with specific mutations of BRCA1 and BRCA2 among Ashkenazi Jews. N Engl J Med 1997;336:1401–8.

16. Warner E, Foulkes W, Goodwin P, et al. Prevalence and penetrance of BRCA1 and BRCA2 gene mutations in unselected Ashkenazi Jewish women with breast cancer. J Natl Cancer Inst 1999;91:1241–7.

17. Thorlacius S, Struewing JP, Hartge P, et al. Population-based study of risk of breast cancer in carriers of BRCA2 mutation. Lancet 1998;352:1337–9.

18. Chen S, Parmigiani G. Meta-analysis of BRCA1 and BRCA2 penetrance. J Clin Oncol 2007;25:1329–33.

19. Martin AM, Weber BL. Genetic and hormonal risk factors in breast cancer. J Natl Cancer Inst 2000;92:1126–35.

20. Kennedy RD, Quinn JE, Johnston PG, Harkin DP. BRCA1: mechanisms of inactivation and implications for management of patients. Lancet 2002;360:1007–14.

21. Easton DF, Ford D, Bishop DT. Breast and ovarian cancer incidence in BRCA1-mutation carriers. Breast Cancer Linkage Consortium. Am J Hum Genet 1995;56:265–71.

22. Struewing JP, Tarone RE, Brody LC, Li FP, Boice JD Jr. BRCA1 mutations in young women with breast cancer. Lancet 1996;347:1493.

23. Hall JM, Lee MK, Newman B, et al. Linkage of early-onset familial breast cancer to chromosome 17q21. Science 1990;250:1684–9.

24. Miki Y, Swensen J, Shattuck-Eidens D, et al. A strong candidate for the breast and ovarian cancer susceptibility gene BRCA1. Science 1994;266:66–71.

25. Walsh T, Casadei S, Coats KH, et al. Spectrum of mutations in BRCA1, BRCA2, CHEK2, and TP53 in families at high risk of breast cancer. JAMA 2006;295:1379–88.

26. Futreal PA, Liu Q, Shattuck-Eidens D, et al. BRCA1 mutations in primary breast and ovarian carcinomas. Science 1994;266:120–2.

27. Castilla LH, Couch FJ, Erdos MR, et al. Mutations in the BRCA1 gene in families with early-onset breast and ovarian cancer. Nat Genet 1994;8:387–91.

28. Friedman LS, Ostermeyer EA, Szabo CI, et al. Confirmation of BRCA1 by analysis of germline mutations linked to breast and ovarian cancer in ten families. Nat Genet 1994;8:399–404.

29. Simard J, Tonin P, Durocher F, et al. Common origins of BRCA1 mutations in Canadian breast and ovarian cancer families. Nat Genet 1994;8:392–8.

30. FitzGerald MG, MacDonald DJ, Krainer M, et al. Germ-line BRCA1 mutations in Jewish and non-Jewish women with early-onset breast cancer. N Engl J Med 1996;334:143–9.

31. Muto MG, Cramer DW, Tangir J, Berkowitz R, Mok S. Frequency of the BRCA1 185delAG mutation among Jewish women with ovarian cancer and matched population controls. Cancer Res 1996;56:1250–2.

32. Abeliovich D, Kaduri L, Lerer I, et al. The founder mutations 185delAG and 5382insC in BRCA1 and 6174delT in BRCA2 appear in 60% of ovarian cancer and 30% of early-onset breast cancer patients among Ashkenazi women. Am J Hum Genet 1997;60:505–14.

33. Couch FJ, Weber BL. Mutations and polymorphisms in the familial early-onset breast cancer (BRCA1) gene. Breast Cancer Information Core. Hum Mutat 1996;8:8–18.

34. Tonin P, Serova O, Lenoir G, et al. BRCA1 mutations in Ashkenazi Jewish women. Am J Hum Genet 1995;57:189.
35. Roa BB, Boyd AA, Volcik K, Richards CS. Ashkenazi Jewish population frequencies for common mutations in BRCA1 and BRCA2. Nat Genet 1996;14:185–7.
36. Berman DB, Wagner-Costalas J, Schultz DC, Lynch HT, Daly M, Godwin AK. Two distinct origins of a common BRCA1 mutation in breast-ovarian cancer families: a genetic study of 15 185delAG-mutation kindreds. Am J Hum Genet 1996;58:1166–76.
37. Offit K, Gilewski T, McGuire P, et al. Germline BRCA1 185delAG mutations in Jewish women with breast cancer. Lancet 1996;347:1643–5.
38. Shen SX, Weaver Z, Xu X, et al. A targeted disruption of the murine Brca1 gene causes gamma-irradiation hypersensitivity and genetic instability. Oncogene 1998;17: 3115–24.
39. Xu X, Qiao W, Linke SP, et al. Genetic interactions between tumor suppressors Brca1 and p53 in apoptosis, cell cycle and tumorigenesis. Nat Genet 2001;28:266–71.
40. Ohta T, Fukuda M. Ubiquitin and breast cancer. Oncogene 2004;23:2079–88.
41. Pavelic K, Gall-Troselj K. Recent advances in molecular genetics of breast cancer. J Mol Med 2001;79:566–73.
42. Zheng L, Li S, Boyer TG, Lee WH. Lessons learned from BRCA1 and BRCA2. Oncogene 2000;19:6159–75.
43. Xu X, Weaver Z, Linke SP, et al. Centrosome amplification and a defective G2-M cell cycle checkpoint induce genetic instability in BRCA1 exon 11 isoform-deficient cells. Mol Cell 1999;3:389–95.
44. Anderson SF, Schlegel BP, Nakajima T, Wolpin ES, Parvin JD. BRCA1 protein is linked to the RNA polymerase II holoenzyme complex via RNA helicase A. Nat Genet 1998;19:254–6.
45. Scully R, Anderson SF, Chao DM, et al. BRCA1 is a component of the RNA polymerase II holoenzyme. Proc Natl Acad Sci U S A 1997;94:5605–10.
46. Scully R, Chen J, Plug A, et al. Association of BRCA1 with Rad51 in mitotic and meiotic cells. Cell 1997;88:265–75.
47. Chen JJ, Silver D, Cantor S, Livingston DM, Scully R. BRCA1, BRCA2, and Rad51 operate in a common DNA damage response pathway. Cancer Res 1999;59:1752s–6s.
48. Hsu LC, White RL. BRCA1 is associated with the centrosome during mitosis. Proc Natl Acad Sci U S A 1998;95:12983–8.
49. Carroll PE, Okuda M, Horn HF, et al. Centrosome hyperamplification in human cancer: chromosome instability induced by p53 mutation and/or Mdm2 overexpression. Oncogene 1999;18:1935–44.
50. Shao N, Chai YL, Shyam E, Reddy P, Rao VN. Induction of apoptosis by the tumor suppressor protein BRCA1. Oncogene 1996;13:1–7.
51. Harkin DP, Bean JM, Miklos D, et al. Induction of GADD45 and JNK/SAPK-dependent apoptosis following inducible expression of BRCA1. Cell 1999;97:575–86.
52. Gowen LC, Avrutskaya AV, Latour AM, Koller BH, Leadon SA. BRCA1 required for transcription-coupled repair of oxidative DNA damage. Science 1998;281:1009–12.
53. Abbott DW, Thompson ME, Robinson-Benion C, Tomlinson G, Jensen RA, Holt JT. BRCA1 expression restores radiation resistance in BRCA1-defective cancer cells through enhancement of transcription-coupled DNA repair. J Biol Chem 1999;274:18808–12.
54. Deng CX, Scott F. Role of the tumor suppressor gene Brca1 in genetic stability and mammary gland tumor formation. Oncogene 2000;19:1059–64.
55. Deng CX, Brodie SG. Roles of BRCA1 and its interacting proteins. Bioessays 2000;22:728–37.
56. Venkitaraman AR. Cancer susceptibility and the functions of BRCA1 and BRCA2. Cell 2002;108:171–82.
57. Deng CX. Tumor formation in Brca1 conditional mutant mice. Environ Mol Mutagen 2002;39:171–7.
58. Brodie SG, Deng CX. BRCA1-associated tumorigenesis: what have we learned from knockout mice? Trends Genet 2001;17:S18–22.

59. Deng CX. BRCA1: cell cycle checkpoint, genetic instability, DNA damage response and cancer evolution. Nucleic Acids Res 2006;34:1416–26.
60. Shamoo Y. Structural insights into BRCA2 function. Curr Opin Struct Biol 2003;13:206–11.
61. Vaughn JP, Cirisano FD, Huper G, et al. Cell cycle control of BRCA2. Cancer Res 1996;56:4590–4.
62. Phelan CM, Lancaster JM, Tonin P, et al. Mutation analysis of the BRCA2 gene in 49 site-specific breast cancer families. Nat Genet 1996;13:120–2.
63. Wooster R, Bignell G, Lancaster J, et al. Identification of the breast cancer susceptibility gene BRCA2. Nature 1995;378:789–92.
64. Tavtigian SV, Simard J, Rommens J, et al. The complete BRCA2 gene and mutations in chromosome 13q-linked kindreds. Nat Genet 1996;12:333–7.
65. Couch FJ, Farid LM, DeShano ML, et al. BRCA2 germline mutations in male breast cancer cases and breast cancer families. Nat Genet 1996;13:123–5.
66. Neuhausen S, Gilewski T, Norton L, et al. Recurrent BRCA2 6174delT mutations in Ashkenazi Jewish women affected by breast cancer. Nat Genet 1996;13:126–8.
67. Lancaster JM, Wooster R, Mangion J, et al. BRCA2 mutations in primary breast and ovarian cancers. Nat Genet 1996;13:238–40.
68. Miki Y, Katagiri T, Kasumi F, Yoshimoto T, Nakamura Y. Mutation analysis in the BRCA2 gene in primary breast cancers. Nat Genet 1996;13:245–7.
69. Takahashi H, Chiu HC, Bandera CA, et al. Mutations of the BRCA2 gene in ovarian carcinomas. Cancer Res 1996;56:2738–41.
70. Agnarsson BA, Jonasson JG, Bjornsdottir IB, Barkardottir RB, Egilsson V, Sigurdsson H. Inherited BRCA2 mutation associated with high grade breast cancer. Breast Cancer Res Treat 1998;47:121–7.
71. Schubert EL, Lee MK, Mefford HC, et al. BRCA2 in American families with four or more cases of breast or ovarian cancer: recurrent and novel mutations, variable expression, penetrance, and the possibility of families whose cancer is not attributable to BRCA1 or BRCA2. Am J Hum Genet 1997;60:1031–40.
72. Inoue R, Ushijima T, Fukutomi T, et al. BRCA2 germline mutations in Japanese breast cancer families. Int J Cancer 1997;74:199–204.
73. Oddoux C, Struewing JP, Clayton CM, et al. The carrier frequency of the BRCA2 6174delT mutation among Ashkenazi Jewish individuals is approximately 1%. Nat Genet 1996;14:188–90.
74. Johannesdottir G, Gudmundsson J, Bergthorsson JT, et al. High prevalence of the 999del5 mutation in Icelandic breast and ovarian cancer patients. Cancer Res 1996;56:3663–5.
75. Vehmanen P, Friedman LS, Eerola H, et al. A low proportion of BRCA2 mutations in Finnish breast cancer families. Am J Hum Genet 1997;60:1050–8.
76. Szabo CI, King MC. Population genetics of BRCA1 and BRCA2. Am J Hum Genet 1997;60:1013–20.
77. Zheng L, Annab LA, Afshari CA, Lee WH, Boyer TG. BRCA1 mediates ligand-independent transcriptional repression of the estrogen receptor. Proc Natl Acad Sci U S A 2001;98:9587–92.
78. Yang Q, Khoury MJ, Rodriguez C, Calle EE, Tatham LM, Flanders WD. Family history score as a predictor of breast cancer mortality: prospective data from the Cancer Prevention Study II, United States, 1982–1991. Am J Epidemiol 1998;147:652–9.
79. Pharoah PD, Day NE, Duffy S, Easton DF, Ponder BA. Family history and the risk of breast cancer: a systematic review and meta-analysis. Int J Cancer 1997;71:800–9.
80. Claus EB, Schildkraut JM, Thompson WD, Risch NJ. The genetic attributable risk of breast and ovarian cancer. Cancer 1996;77:2318–24.
81. Familial breast cancer: collaborative reanalysis of individual data from 52 epidemiological studies including 58,209 women with breast cancer and 101,986 women without the disease. Lancet 2001;358:1389–99.
82. Beers NS, Kemeny A, Sherritt L, Palfrey JS. Variations in state-level definitions: children with special health care needs. Public Health Rep 2003;118:434–47.

83. Ford D, Easton DF, Peto J. Estimates of the gene frequency of BRCA1 and its contribution to breast and ovarian cancer incidence. Am J Hum Genet 1995;57:1457–62.
84. Risch HA, McLaughlin JR, Cole DE, et al. Population BRCA1 and BRCA2 mutation frequencies and cancer penetrances: a kin-cohort study in Ontario, Canada. J Natl Cancer Inst 2006;98:1694–706.
85. Antoniou AC, Pharoah PD, McMullan G, et al. A comprehensive model for familial breast cancer incorporating BRCA1, BRCA2 and other genes. Br J Cancer 2002;86:76–83.
86. Whittemore AS, Gong G, John EM, et al. Prevalence of BRCA1 mutation carriers among U.S. non-Hispanic Whites. Cancer Epidemiol Biomarkers Prev 2004;13:2078–83.
87. Tonin P, Weber B, Offit K, et al. Frequency of recurrent BRCA1 and BRCA2 mutations in Ashkenazi Jewish breast cancer families. Nat Med 1996;2:1179–83.
88. Verhoog LC, van den Ouweland AM, Berns E, et al. Large regional differences in the frequency of distinct BRCA1/BRCA2 mutations in 517 Dutch breast and/or ovarian cancer families. Eur J Cancer 2001;37:2082–90.
89. Gorski B, Jakubowska A, Huzarski T, et al. A high proportion of founder BRCA1 mutations in Polish breast cancer families. Int J Cancer 2004;110:683–6.
90. Dite GS, Jenkins MA, Southey MC, et al. Familial risks, early-onset breast cancer, and BRCA1 and BRCA2 germline mutations. J Natl Cancer Inst 2003;95:448–57.
91. Feuer EJ, Wun LM, Boring CC, Flanders WD, Timmel MJ, Tong T. The lifetime risk of developing breast cancer. J Natl Cancer Inst 1993;85:892–7.
92. Rockhill B, Weinberg CR, Newman B. Population attributable fraction estimation for established breast cancer risk factors: considering the issues of high prevalence and unmodifiability. Am J Epidemiol 1998;147:826–33.
93. Madigan MP, Ziegler RG, Benichou J, Byrne C, Hoover RN. Proportion of breast cancer cases in the United States explained by well-established risk factors. J Natl Cancer Inst 1995;87:1681–5.
94. Gail MH, Brinton LA, Byar DP, et al. Projecting individualized probabilities of developing breast cancer for white females who are being examined annually. J Natl Cancer Inst 1989;81:1879–86.
95. Hildreth NG, Shore RE, Dvoretsky PM. The risk of breast cancer after irradiation of the thymus in infancy. N Engl J Med 1989;321:1281–4.
96. Hunter DJ, Spiegelman D, Adami HO, et al. Cohort studies of fat intake and the risk of breast cancer-a pooled analysis. N Engl J Med 1996;334:356–61.
97. Rosenberg L, Palmer JR, Rao RS, et al. Case-control study of oral contraceptive use and risk of breast cancer. Am J Epidemiol 1996;143:25–37.
98. Michels KB, Willett WC. Does induced or spontaneous abortion affect the risk of breast cancer? Epidemiology 1996;7:521–8.
99. Antoniou AC, Shenton A, Maher ER, et al. Parity and breast cancer risk among BRCA1 and BRCA2 mutation carriers. Breast Cancer Res 2006;8:R72.
100. Andrieu N, Goldgar DE, Easton DF, et al. Pregnancies, breast-feeding, and breast cancer risk in the International BRCA1/2 Carrier Cohort Study (IBCCS). J Natl Cancer Inst 2006;98:535–44.
101. Chang-Claude J, Andrieu N, Rookus M, et al. Age at menarche and menopause and breast cancer risk in the International BRCA1/2 Carrier Cohort Study. Cancer Epidemiol Biomarkers Prev 2007;16:740–6.
102. Spiegelman D, Colditz GA, Hunter D, Hertzmark E. Validation of the Gail et al. model for predicting individual breast cancer risk. J Natl Cancer Inst 1994;86:600–7.
103. Bondy ML, Lustbader ED, Halabi S, Ross E, Vogel VG. Validation of a breast cancer risk assessment model in women with a positive family history. J Natl Cancer Inst 1994;86:620–5.
104. Costantino JP, Gail MH, Pee D, et al. Validation studies for models projecting the risk of invasive and total breast cancer incidence. J Natl Cancer Inst 1999;91:1541–8.
105. Rockhill B, Spiegelman D, Byrne C, Hunter DJ, Colditz GA. Validation of the Gail et al. model of breast cancer risk prediction and implications for chemoprevention. J Natl Cancer Inst 2001;93:358–66.

106. Decarli A, Calza S, Masala G, Specchia C, Palli D, Gail MH. Gail model for prediction of absolute risk of invasive breast cancer: independent evaluation in the Florence-European Prospective Investigation into Cancer and Nutrition cohort. J Natl Cancer Inst 2006;98:1686–93.

107. Chen J, Pee D, Ayyagari R, et al. Projecting absolute invasive breast cancer risk in white women with a model that includes mammographic density. J Natl Cancer Inst 2006;98:1215–26.

108. Barlow WE, White E, Ballard-Barbash R, et al. Prospective breast cancer risk prediction model for women undergoing screening mammography. J Natl Cancer Inst 2006;98:1204–14.

109. Mitchell G, Antoniou AC, Warren R, et al. Mammographic density and breast cancer risk in BRCA1 and BRCA2 mutation carriers. Cancer Res 2006;66:1866–72.

110. Claus EB, Risch N, Thompson WD. Autosomal dominant inheritance of early-onset breast cancer. Implications for risk prediction. Cancer 1994;73:643–51.

111. Saslow D, Boetes C, Burke W, et al. American Cancer Society guidelines for breast screening with MRI as an adjunct to mammography. CA Cancer J Clin 2007;57:75–89.

112. Simon MS, Korczak JF, Yee CL, et al. Breast cancer risk estimates for relatives of white and African American women with breast cancer in the Women's Contraceptive and Reproductive Experiences Study. J Clin Oncol 2006;24:2498–504.

113. Claus EB, Risch N, Thompson WD. Genetic analysis of breast cancer in the cancer and steroid hormone study. Am J Hum Genet 1991;48:232–42.

114. Couch FJ, DeShano ML, Blackwood MA, et al. BRCA1 mutations in women attending clinics that evaluate the risk of breast cancer. N Engl J Med 1997;336:1409–15.

115. Shattuck-Eidens D, Oliphant A, McClure M, et al. BRCA1 sequence analysis in women at high risk for susceptibility mutations. Risk factor analysis and implications for genetic testing. JAMA 1997;278:1242–50.

116. Berry DA, Parmigiani G, Sanchez J, Schildkraut J, Winer E. Probability of carrying a mutation of breast-ovarian cancer gene BRCA1 based on family history. J Natl Cancer Inst 1997;89:227–38.

117. Parmigiani G, Berry D, Aguilar O. Determining carrier probabilities for breast cancer-susceptibility genes BRCA1 and BRCA2. Am J Hum Genet 1998;62:145–58.

118. Hartge P, Struewing JP, Wacholder S, Brody LC, Tucker MA. The prevalence of common BRCA1 and BRCA2 mutations among Ashkenazi Jews. Am J Hum Genet 1999;64:963–70.

119. Gilpin CA, Carson N, Hunter AG. A preliminary validation of a family history assessment form to select women at risk for breast or ovarian cancer for referral to a genetics center. Clin Genet 2000;58:299–308.

120. Vahteristo P, Eerola H, Tamminen A, Blomqvist C, Nevanlinna H. A probability model for predicting BRCA1 and BRCA2 mutations in breast and breast-ovarian cancer families. Br J Cancer 2001;84:704–8.

121. Frank TS, Deffenbaugh AM, Reid JE, et al. Clinical characteristics of individuals with germline mutations in BRCA1 and BRCA2: analysis of 10,000 individuals. J Clin Oncol 2002;20:1480–90.

122. Apicella C, Dowty JG, Dite GS, et al. Validation study of the LAMBDA model for predicting the BRCA1 or BRCA2 mutation carrier status of North American Ashkenazi Jewish women. Clin Genet 2007;72:87–97.

123. de la Hoya M, Diez O, Perez-Segura P, et al. Pre-test prediction models of BRCA1 or BRCA2 mutation in breast/ovarian families attending familial cancer clinics. J Med Genet 2003;40:503–10.

124. Evans DG, Eccles DM, Rahman N, et al. A new scoring system for the chances of identifying a BRCA1/2 mutation outperforms existing models including BRCAPRO. J Med Genet 2004;41:474–80.

125. Antoniou AC, Pharoah PP, Smith P, Easton DF. The BOADICEA model of genetic susceptibility to breast and ovarian cancer. Br J Cancer 2004;91:1580–90.

126. Tyrer J, Duffy SW, Cuzick J. A breast cancer prediction model incorporating familial and personal risk factors. Stat Med 2004;23:1111–30.

127. Parmigiani G, Chen S, Iversen ES Jr.,et al.., Validity of models for predicting BRCA1 and BRCA2 mutations. Ann Intern Med 2007;147:441–50.
128. Domchek SM, Eisen A, Calzone K, Stopfer J, Blackwood A, Weber BL. Application of breast cancer risk prediction models in clinical practice. J Clin Oncol 2003;21:593–601.
129. Trepanier A, Ahrens M, McKinnon W, et al. Genetic cancer risk assessment and counseling: recommendations of the national society of genetic counselors. J Genet Couns 2004;13:83–114.
130. American Society of Clinical Oncology policy statement update: genetic testing for cancer susceptibility. J Clin Oncol 2003;21:2397–406.
131. Nanda R, Schumm LP, Cummings S, et al. Genetic testing in an ethnically diverse cohort of high-risk women: a comparative analysis of BRCA1 and BRCA2 mutations in American families of European and African ancestry. JAMA 2005;294:1925–33.
132. Vogel KJ, Atchley DP, Erlichman J, et al. BRCA1 and BRCA2 genetic testing in Hispanic patients: mutation prevalence and evaluation of the BRCAPRO risk assessment model. J Clin Oncol 2007;25:4635–41.
133. Berliner JL, Fay AM. Risk assessment and genetic counseling for hereditary breast and ovarian cancer: recommendations of the National Society of Genetic Counselors. J Genet Couns 2007;16:241–60.
134. Weitzel JN, Lagos VI, Cullinane CA, et al. Limited family structure and BRCA gene mutation status in single cases of breast cancer. JAMA 2007;297:2587–95.
135. Braithwaite D, Emery J, Walter F, Prevost AT, Sutton S. Psychological impact of genetic counseling for familial cancer: a systematic review and meta-analysis. J Natl Cancer Inst 2004;96:122–33.
136. Lerman C, Narod S, Schulman K, et al. BRCA1 testing in families with hereditary breast-ovarian cancer. A prospective study of patient decision making and outcomes. JAMA 1996;275:1885–92.
137. Biesecker BB, Ishibe N, Hadley DW, et al. Psychosocial factors predicting BRCA1/BRCA2 testing decisions in members of hereditary breast and ovarian cancer families. Am J Med Genet 2000;93:257–63.
138. Botkin JR, Smith KR, Croyle RT, et al. Genetic testing for a BRCA1 mutation: prophylactic surgery and screening behavior in women 2 years post testing. Am J Med Genet A 2003;118:201–9.
139. Schneider KA. Genetic counseling for BRCA1/BRCA2 testing. Genet Test 1997;1:91–8.
140. Armstrong K, Weber B, FitzGerald G, et al. Life insurance and breast cancer risk assessment: adverse selection, genetic testing decisions, and discrimination. Am J Med Genet A 2003;120:359–64.
141. Matloff ET, Shappell H, Brierley K, Bernhardt BA, McKinnon W, Peshkin BN. What would you do? Specialists' perspectives on cancer genetic testing, prophylactic surgery, and insurance discrimination. J Clin Oncol 2000;18:2484–92.
142. Hudson KL. Prohibiting genetic discrimination. N Engl J Med 2007;356:2021–3.
143. Statement of the American Society of Clinical Oncology: genetic testing for cancer susceptibility, Adopted on February 20, 1996. J Clin Oncol 1996;14:1730–6; 0072.
144. Berry DA, Iversen ES Jr., Gudbjartsson DF, et al. BRCAPRO validation, sensitivity of genetic testing of BRCA1/BRCA2, and prevalence of other breast cancer susceptibility genes. J Clin Oncol 2002;20:2701–12.
145. Brekelmans CT, Seynaeve C, Bartels CC, et al. Effectiveness of breast cancer surveillance in BRCA1/2 gene mutation carriers and women with high familial risk. J Clin Oncol 2001;19:924–30.
146. Kriege M, Brekelmans CT, Boetes C, et al. Efficacy of MRI and mammography for breast-cancer screening in women with a familial or genetic predisposition. N Engl J Med 2004;351:427–37.
147. Scheuer L, Kauff N, Robson M, et al. Outcome of preventive surgery and screening for breast and ovarian cancer in BRCA mutation carriers. J Clin Oncol 2002;20:1260–8.
148. Warner E, Plewes DB, Hill KA, et al. Surveillance of BRCA1 and BRCA2 mutation carriers with magnetic resonance imaging, ultrasound, mammography, and clinical breast examination. JAMA 2004;292:1317–25.

149. Hackshaw AK, Paul EA. Breast self-examination and death from breast cancer: a meta-analysis. Br J Cancer 2003;88:1047–53.
150. Tilanus-Linthorst MM, Obdeijn IM, Bartels KC, de Koning HJ, Oudkerk M. First experiences in screening women at high risk for breast cancer with MR imaging. Breast Cancer Res Treat 2000;63:53–60.
151. Ziv E, Shepherd J, Smith-Bindman R, Kerlikowske K. Mammographic breast density and family history of breast cancer. J Natl Cancer Inst 2003;95:556–8.
152. Buist DS, Porter PL, Lehman C, Taplin SH, White E. Factors contributing to mammography failure in women aged 40–49 years. J Natl Cancer Inst 2004;96:1432–40.
153. Kerlikowske K, Grady D, Barclay J, Sickles EA, Ernster V. Effect of age, breast density, and family history on the sensitivity of first screening mammography. JAMA 1996;276:33–8.
154. Collett K, Stefansson IM, Eide J, et al. A basal epithelial phenotype is more frequent in interval breast cancers compared with screen detected tumors. Cancer Epidemiol Biomarkers Prev 2005;14:1108–12.
155. Pisano ED, Gatsonis C, Hendrick E, et al. Diagnostic performance of digital versus film mammography for breast-cancer screening. N Engl J Med 2005;353:1773–83.
156. Ronckers CM, Erdmann CA, Land CE. Radiation and breast cancer: a review of current evidence. Breast Cancer Res 2005;7:21–32.
157. Andrieu N, Easton DF, Chang-Claude J, et al. Effect of chest X-rays on the risk of breast cancer among BRCA1/2 mutation carriers in the international BRCA1/2 carrier cohort study: a report from the EMBRACE, GENEPSO, GEO-HEBON, and IBCCS Collaborators' Group. J Clin Oncol 2006;24:3361–6.
158. Kuhl CK, Schmutzler RK, Leutner CC, et al. Breast MR imaging screening in 192 women proved or suspected to be carriers of a breast cancer susceptibility gene: preliminary results. Radiology 2000;215:267–79.
159. Warner E, Plewes DB, Shumak RS, et al. Comparison of breast magnetic resonance imaging, mammography, and ultrasound for surveillance of women at high risk for hereditary breast cancer. J Clin Oncol 2001;19:3524–31.
160. Podo F, Sardanelli F, Canese R, et al. The Italian multi-centre project on evaluation of MRI and other imaging modalities in early detection of breast cancer in subjects at high genetic risk. J Exp Clin Cancer Res 2002;21:115–24.
161. Leach MO, Boggis CR, Dixon AK, et al. Screening with magnetic resonance imaging and mammography of a UK population at high familial risk of breast cancer: a prospective multicentre cohort study (MARIBS). Lancet 2005;365:1769–78.
162. Kuhl CK, Schrading S, Leutner CC, et al. Mammography, breast ultrasound, and magnetic resonance imaging for surveillance of women at high familial risk for breast cancer. J Clin Oncol 2005;23:8469–76.
163. Stoutjesdijk MJ, Boetes C, Jager GJ, et al. Magnetic resonance imaging and mammography in women with a hereditary risk of breast cancer. J Natl Cancer Inst 2001;93:1095–102.
164. Morris EA, Liberman L, Ballon DJ, et al. MRI of occult breast carcinoma in a high-risk population. AJR Am J Roentgenol 2003;181:619–26.
165. Sardanelli F, Podo F. Breast MR imaging in women at high-risk of breast cancer. Is something changing in early breast cancer detection? Eur Radiol 2007;17:873–87.
166. Morakkabati-Spitz N, Leutner C, Schild H, Traeber F, Kuhl C. Diagnostic usefulness of segmental and linear enhancement in dynamic breast MRI. Eur Radiol 2005;15: 2010–7.
167. Kuhl CK, Schrading S, Bieling HB, et al. MRI for diagnosis of pure ductal carcinoma in situ: a prospective observational study. Lancet 2007;370:485–92.
168. Robson M, Offit K. Clinical practice. Management of an inherited predisposition to breast cancer. N Engl J Med 2007;357:154–62.
169. Robson ME, Offit K. Breast MRI for women with hereditary cancer risk. JAMA 2004;292:1368–70.
170. Lehman CD, Blume JD, Weatherall P, et al. Screening women at high risk for breast cancer with mammography and magnetic resonance imaging. Cancer 2005;103:1898–905.
171. Lord SJ, Irwig L, Simes RJ. When is measuring sensitivity and specificity sufficient to evaluate a diagnostic test, and when do we need randomized trials? Ann Intern Med 2006;144:850–5.

172. Hermsen BB, Olivier RI, Verheijen RH, et al. No efficacy of annual gynaecological screening in BRCA1/2 mutation carriers; an observational follow-up study. Br J Cancer 2007;96:1335–42.

173. Olivier RI, Lubsen-Brandsma MA, Verhoef S, van Beurden M. CA125 and transvaginal ultrasound monitoring in high-risk women cannot prevent the diagnosis of advanced ovarian cancer. Gynecol Oncol 2006;100:20–6.

174. Hartmann LC, Schaid DJ, Woods JE, et al. Efficacy of bilateral prophylactic mastectomy in women with a family history of breast cancer. N Engl J Med 1999;340:77–84.

175. Hartmann LC, Sellers TA, Schaid DJ, et al. Efficacy of bilateral prophylactic mastectomy in BRCA1 and BRCA2 gene mutation carriers. J Natl Cancer Inst 2001;93:1633–7.

176. Meijers-Heijboer H, van Geel B, van Putten WL, et al. Breast cancer after prophylactic bilateral mastectomy in women with a BRCA1 or BRCA2 mutation. N Engl J Med 2001;345:159–64.

177. Rebbeck TR, Friebel T, Lynch HT, et al. Bilateral prophylactic mastectomy reduces breast cancer risk in BRCA1 and BRCA2 mutation carriers: the PROSE Study Group. J Clin Oncol 2004;22:1055–62.

178. Herrinton LJ, Barlow WE, Yu O, et al. Efficacy of prophylactic mastectomy in women with unilateral breast cancer: a cancer research network project. J Clin Oncol 2005;23:4275–86.

179. Pennisi VR, Capozzi A. Subcutaneous mastectomy data: a final statistical analysis of 1500 patients. Aesthetic Plast Surg 1989;13:15–21.

180. Hartmann LC, Degnim A, Schaid DJ. Prophylactic mastectomy for BRCA1/2 carriers: progress and more questions. J Clin Oncol 2004;22:981–3.

181. Guillem JG, Wood WC, Moley JF, et al. ASCO/SSO review of current role of risk-reducing surgery in common hereditary cancer syndromes. J Clin Oncol 2006;24:4642–60.

182. Finch A, Beiner M, Lubinski J, et al. Salpingo-oophorectomy and the risk of ovarian, fallopian tube, and peritoneal cancers in women with a BRCA1 or BRCA2 Mutation. JAMA 2006;296:185–92.

183. Kauff ND, Satagopan JM, Robson ME, et al. Risk-reducing salpingo-oophorectomy in women with a BRCA1 or BRCA2 mutation. N Engl J Med 2002;346:1609–15.

184. Rebbeck TR, Lynch HT, Neuhausen SL, et al. Prophylactic oophorectomy in carriers of BRCA1 or BRCA2 mutations. N Engl J Med 2002;346:1616–22.

185. Eisen A, Lubinski J, Klijn J, et al. Breast cancer risk following bilateral oophorectomy in BRCA1 and BRCA2 mutation carriers: an international case-control study. J Clin Oncol 2005;23:7491–6.

186. Domchek SM, Friebel TM, Neuhausen SL, et al. Mortality after bilateral salpingo-oophorectomy in BRCA1 and BRCA2 mutation carriers: a prospective cohort study. Lancet Oncol 2006;7:223–9.

187. Casey MJ, Synder C, Bewtra C, Narod SA, Watson P, Lynch HT. Intra-abdominal carcinomatosis after prophylactic oophorectomy in women of hereditary breast ovarian cancer syndrome kindreds associated with BRCA1 and BRCA2 mutations. Gynecol Oncol 2005;97:457–67.

188. Rebbeck TR, Friebel T, Wagner T, et al. Effect of short-term hormone replacement therapy on breast cancer risk reduction after bilateral prophylactic oophorectomy in BRCA1 and BRCA2 mutation carriers: the PROSE Study Group. J Clin Oncol 2005;23:7804–10.

189. Fisher B, Costantino JP, Wickerham DL, et al. Tamoxifen for prevention of breast cancer: report of the National Surgical Adjuvant Breast and Bowel Project P-1 Study. J Natl Cancer Inst 1998;90:1371–88.

190. King MC, Wieand S, Hale K, et al. Tamoxifen and breast cancer incidence among women with inherited mutations in BRCA1 and BRCA2: National Surgical Adjuvant Breast and Bowel Project (NSABP-P1) Breast Cancer Prevention Trial. JAMA 2001;286:2251–6.

191. Narod SA, Brunet JS, Ghadirian P, et al. Tamoxifen and risk of contralateral breast cancer in BRCA1 and BRCA2 mutation carriers: a case-control study. Hereditary Breast Cancer Clinical Study Group. Lancet 2000;356:1876–81.

192. Pierce LJ, Levin AM, Rebbeck TR, et al. Ten-year multi-institutional results of breast-conserving surgery and radiotherapy in BRCA1/2-associated stage I/II breast cancer. J Clin Oncol 2006;24:2437–43.
193. Gronwald J, Tung N, Foulkes WD, et al. Tamoxifen and contralateral breast cancer in BRCA1 and BRCA2 carriers: an update. Int J Cancer 2006;118:2281–4.
194. Metcalfe K, Lynch HT, Ghadirian P, et al. Contralateral breast cancer in BRCA1 and BRCA2 mutation carriers. J Clin Oncol 2004;22:2328–35.
195. Foulkes WD, Goffin J, Brunet JS, Begin LR, Wong N, Chappuis PO. Tamoxifen may be an effective adjuvant treatment for BRCA1-related breast cancer irrespective of estrogen receptor status. J Natl Cancer Inst 2002;94:1504–6.
196. Vogel VG, Costantino JP, Wickerham DL, et al. Effects of tamoxifen vs raloxifene on the risk of developing invasive breast cancer and other disease outcomes: the NSABP Study of Tamoxifen and Raloxifene (STAR) P-2 trial. JAMA 2006;295:2727–41.
197. Premkumar A, Venzon DJ, Avila N, et al. Gynecologic and hormonal effects of raloxifene in premenopausal women. Fertil Steril 2007;88:1637–1644.
198. Narod SA, Risch H, Moslehi R, et al. Oral contraceptives and the risk of hereditary ovarian cancer. Hereditary Ovarian Cancer Clinical Study Group. N Engl J Med 1998;339:424–8.
199. McLaughlin JR, Risch HA, Lubinski J, et al. Reproductive risk factors for ovarian cancer in carriers of BRCA1 or BRCA2 mutations: a case-control study. Lancet Oncol 2007;8:26–34.
200. Modan B, Hartge P, Hirsh-Yechezkel G, et al. Parity, oral contraceptives, and the risk of ovarian cancer among carriers and noncarriers of a BRCA1 or BRCA2 mutation. N Engl J Med 2001;345:235–40.
201. Whittemore AS, Balise RR, Pharoah PD, et al. Oral contraceptive use and ovarian cancer risk among carriers of BRCA1 or BRCA2 mutations. Br J Cancer 2004;91:1911–5.
202. Haile RW, Thomas DC, McGuire V, et al. BRCA1 and BRCA2 mutation carriers, oral contraceptive use, and breast cancer before age 50. Cancer Epidemiol Biomarkers Prev 2006;15:1863–70.
203. Narod SA, Dube MP, Klijn J, et al. Oral contraceptives and the risk of breast cancer in BRCA1 and BRCA2 mutation carriers. J Natl Cancer Inst 2002;94:1773–9.
204. Brohet RM, Goldgar DE, Easton DF, et al. Oral contraceptives and breast cancer risk in the international BRCA1/2 carrier cohort study: a report from EMBRACE, GENEPSO, GEO-HEBON, and the IBCCS Collaborating Group. J Clin Oncol 2007;25:3831–6.
205. Arason A, Barkardottir RB, Egilsson V. Linkage analysis of chromosome 17q markers and breast-ovarian cancer in Icelandic families, and possible relationship to prostatic cancer. Am J Hum Genet 1993;52:711–7.
206. Anderson DE, Badzioch MD. Familial breast cancer risks. Effects of prostate and other cancers. Cancer 1993;72:114–9.
207. Nelson CL, Sellers TA, Rich SS, Potter JD, McGovern PG, Kushi LH. Familial clustering of colon, breast, uterine, and ovarian cancers as assessed by family history. Genet Epidemiol 1993;10:235–44.
208. Foulkes WD, Metcalfe K, Hanna W, et al. Disruption of the expected positive correlation between breast tumor size and lymph node status in BRCA1-related breast carcinoma. Cancer 2003;98:1569–77.
209. Foulkes WD. BRCA1 and BRCA2: chemosensitivity, treatment outcomes and prognosis. Fam Cancer 2006;5:135–42.
210. Beiner ME, Finch A, Rosen B, et al. The risk of endometrial cancer in women with BRCA1 and BRCA2 mutations. A prospective study. Gynecol Oncol 2007;104:7–10.
211. Lakhani SR, Gusterson BA, Jacquemier J, et al. The pathology of familial breast cancer: histological features of cancers in families not attributable to mutations in BRCA1 or BRCA2. Clin Cancer Res 2000;6:782–9.
212. Armes JE, Egan AJ, Southey MC, et al. The histologic phenotypes of breast carcinoma occurring before age 40 years in women with and without BRCA1 or BRCA2 germline mutations: a population-based study. Cancer 1998;83:2335–45.

213. Marcus JN, Watson P, Page DL, et al. Hereditary breast cancer: pathobiology, prognosis, and BRCA1 and BRCA2 gene linkage. Cancer 1996;77:697–709.
214. Marcus JN, Watson P, Page DL, et al. BRCA2 hereditary breast cancer pathophenotype. Breast Cancer Res Treat 1997;44:275–7.
215. Lakhani SR, Jacquemier J, Sloane JP, et al. Multifactorial analysis of differences between sporadic breast cancers and cancers involving BRCA1 and BRCA2 mutations. J Natl Cancer Inst 1998;90:1138–45.
216. Hoogerbrugge N, Bult P, de Widt-Levert LM, et al. High prevalence of premalignant lesions in prophylactically removed breasts from women at hereditary risk for breast cancer. J Clin Oncol 2003;21:41–5.
217. Kauff ND, Brogi E, Scheuer L, et al. Epithelial lesions in prophylactic mastectomy specimens from women with BRCA mutations. Cancer 2003;97:1601–8.
218. Chappuis PO, Donato E, Goffin JR, et al. Cyclin E expression in breast cancer: predicting germline BRCA1 mutations, prognosis and response to treatment. Ann Oncol 2005;16:735–42.
219. Chappuis PO, Kapusta L, Begin LR, et al. Germline BRCA1/2 mutations and p27(Kip1) protein levels independently predict outcome after breast cancer. J Clin Oncol 2000;18:4045–52.
220. Lynch BJ, Holden JA, Buys SS, Neuhausen SL, Gaffney DK. Pathobiologic characteristics of hereditary breast cancer. Hum Pathol 1998;29:1140–4.
221. Quenneville LA, Phillips KA, Ozcelik H, et al. HER-2/neu status and tumor morphology of invasive breast carcinomas in Ashkenazi women with known BRCA1 mutation status in the Ontario Familial Breast Cancer Registry. Cancer 2002;95:2068–75.
222. Goffin JR, Chappuis PO, Begin LR, et al. Impact of germline BRCA1 mutations and overexpression of p53 on prognosis and response to treatment following breast carcinoma: 10-year follow up data. Cancer 2003;97:527–36.
223. Honrado E, Benitez J, Palacios J. Histopathology of BRCA1- and BRCA2-associated breast cancer. Crit Rev Oncol Hematol 2006;59:27–39.
224. Goffin JR, Straume O, Chappuis PO, et al. Glomeruloid microvascular proliferation is associated with p53 expression, germline BRCA1 mutations and an adverse outcome following breast cancer. Br J Cancer 2003;89:1031–4.
225. Grushko TA, Dignam JJ, Das S, et al. MYC is amplified in BRCA1-associated breast cancers. Clin Cancer Res 2004;10:499–507.
226. Adem C, Soderberg CL, Hafner K, et al. ERBB2, TBX2, RPS6KB1, and MYC alterations in breast tissues of BRCA1 and BRCA2 mutation carriers. Genes Chromosomes Cancer 2004;41:1–11.
227. Lakhani SR, Van De Vijver MJ, Jacquemier J, et al. The pathology of familial breast cancer: predictive value of immunohistochemical markers estrogen receptor, progesterone receptor, HER-2, and p53 in patients with mutations in BRCA1 and BRCA2. J Clin Oncol 2002;20:2310–8.
228. Palacios J, Honrado E, Osorio A, et al. Immunohistochemical characteristics defined by tissue microarray of hereditary breast cancer not attributable to BRCA1 or BRCA2 mutations: differences from breast carcinomas arising in BRCA1 and BRCA2 mutation carriers. Clin Cancer Res 2003;9:3606–14.
229. Eerola H, Heikkila P, Tamminen A, Aittomaki K, Blomqvist C, Nevanlinna H. Histopathological features of breast tumours in BRCA1, BRCA2 and mutation-negative breast cancer families. Breast Cancer Res 2005;7:R93–100.
230. Osin P, Gusterson BA, Philp E, et al. Predicted anti-oestrogen resistance in BRCA-associated familial breast cancers. Eur J Cancer 1998;34:1683–6.
231. Eisinger F, Nogues C, Guinebretiere JM, et al. Novel indications for BRCA1 screening using individual clinical and morphological features. Int J Cancer 1999;84:263–7.
232. Noguchi S, Kasugai T, Miki Y, Fukutomi T, Emi M, Nomizu T. Clinicopathologic analysis of BRCA1- or BRCA2-associated hereditary breast carcinoma in Japanese women. Cancer 1999;85:2200–5.
233. Robson ME, Chappuis PO, Satagopan J, et al. A combined analysis of outcome following breast cancer: differences in survival based on BRCA1/BRCA2 mutation status and administration of adjuvant treatment. Breast Cancer Res 2004;6:R8-R17.

234. Oldenburg RA, Kroeze-Jansema K, Meijers-Heijboer H, et al. Characterization of familial non-BRCA1/2 breast tumors by loss of heterozygosity and immunophenotyping. Clin Cancer Res 2006;12:1693–700.
235. Foulkes WD, Metcalfe K, Sun P, et al. Estrogen receptor status in BRCA1- and BRCA2-related breast cancer: the influence of age, grade, and histological type. Clin Cancer Res 2004;10:2029–34.
236. Grushko TA, Blackwood MA, Schumm PL, et al. Molecular-cytogenetic analysis of HER-2/neu gene in BRCA1-associated breast cancers. Cancer Res 2002;62:1481–8.
237. Johannsson OT, Idvall I, Anderson C, et al. Tumour biological features of BRCA1-induced breast and ovarian cancer. Eur J Cancer 1997;33:362–71.
238. Stark GR. Regulation and mechanisms of mammalian gene amplification. Adv Cancer Res 1993;61:87–113.
239. Honrado E, Osorio A, Palacios J, Benitez J. Pathology and gene expression of hereditary breast tumors associated with BRCA1, BRCA2 and CHEK2 gene mutations. Oncogene 2006;25:5837–45.
240. Hedenfalk I, Duggan D, Chen Y, et al. Gene-expression profiles in hereditary breast cancer. N Engl J Med 2001;344:539–48.
241. Vaziri SA, Krumroy LM, Elson P, et al. Breast tumor immunophenotype of BRCA1-mutation carriers is influenced by age at diagnosis. Clin Cancer Res 2001;7:1937–45.
242. Lakhani SR, Reis-Filho JS, Fulford L, et al. Prediction of BRCA1 status in patients with breast cancer using estrogen receptor and basal phenotype. Clin Cancer Res 2005;11:5175–80.
243. Palacios J, Honrado E, Osorio A, Diez O, Rivas C, Benitez J. Re: Germline BRCA1 mutations and a basal epithelial phenotype in breast cancer. J Natl Cancer Inst 2004;96:712–4; author reply 4.
244. Signoretti S, Di Marcotullio L, Richardson A, et al. Oncogenic role of the ubiquitin ligase subunit Skp2 in human breast cancer. J Clin Invest 2002;110:633–41.
245. Fisher B, Anderson S, Bryant J, et al. Twenty-year follow-up of a randomized trial comparing total mastectomy, lumpectomy, and lumpectomy plus irradiation for the treatment of invasive breast cancer. N Engl J Med 2002;347:1233–41.
246. Veronesi U, Cascinelli N, Mariani L, et al. Twenty-year follow-up of a randomized study comparing breast-conserving surgery with radical mastectomy for early breast cancer. N Engl J Med 2002;347:1227–32.
247. Eccles D, Simmonds P, Goddard J, et al. Familial breast cancer: an investigation into the outcome of treatment for early stage disease. Fam Cancer 2001;1:65–72.
248. Robson M, Svahn T, McCormick B, et al. Appropriateness of breast-conserving treatment of breast carcinoma in women with germline mutations in BRCA1 or BRCA2: a clinic-based series. Cancer 2005;103:44–51.
249. Seynaeve C, Verhoog LC, van de Bosch LM, et al. Ipsilateral breast tumour recurrence in hereditary breast cancer following breast-conserving therapy. Eur J Cancer 2004;40:1150–8.
250. Quinn JE, Kennedy RD, Mullan PB, et al. BRCA1 functions as a differential modulator of chemotherapy-induced apoptosis. Cancer Res 2003;63:6221–8.
251. Kennedy RD, Quinn JE, Mullan PB, Johnston PG, Harkin DP. The role of BRCA1 in the cellular response to chemotherapy. J Natl Cancer Inst 2004;96:1659–68.
252. Chappuis PO, Goffin J, Wong N, et al. A significant response to neoadjuvant chemotherapy in BRCA1/2 related breast cancer. J Med Genet 2002;39:608–10.
253. Rouzier R, Perou CM, Symmans WF, et al. Breast cancer molecular subtypes respond differently to preoperative chemotherapy. Clin Cancer Res 2005;11:5678–85.
254. Rubinstein WS. Hereditary breast cancer: pathobiology, clinical translation, and potential for targeted cancer therapeutics. Fam Cancer 2007.
255. Farmer H, McCabe N, Lord CJ, et al. Targeting the DNA repair defect in BRCA mutant cells as a therapeutic strategy. Nature 2005;434:917–21.
256. Bryant HE, Schultz N, Thomas HD, et al. Specific killing of BRCA2-deficient tumours with inhibitors of poly(ADP-ribose) polymerase. Nature 2005;434:913–7.

257. Helleday T, Bryant HE, Schultz N. Poly(ADP-ribose) polymerase (PARP-1) in homologous recombination and as a target for cancer therapy. Cell Cycle 2005;4:1176–8.
258. Szabo G, Bahrle S, Stumpf N, et al. Poly(ADP-Ribose) polymerase inhibition reduces reperfusion injury after heart transplantation. Circ Res 2002;90:100–6.
259. Alano CC, Kauppinen TM, Valls AV, Swanson RA. Minocycline inhibits poly(ADP-ribose) polymerase-1 at nanomolar concentrations. Proc Natl Acad Sci USA 2006;103: 9685–90.
260. Slamon DJ, Clark GM, Wong SG, Levin WJ, Ullrich A, McGuire WL. Human breast cancer: correlation of relapse and survival with amplification of the HER-2/neu oncogene. Science 1987;235:177–82.
261. Verhoog LC, Brekelmans CT, Seynaeve C, et al. Survival in hereditary breast cancer associated with germline mutations of BRCA2. J Clin Oncol 1999;17:3396–402.
262. Rennert G, Bisland-Naggan S, Barnett-Griness O, et al. Clinical outcomes of breast cancer in carriers of BRCA1 and BRCA2 mutations. N Engl J Med 2007;357:115–23.
263. Li FP, Fraumeni JF Jr. Rhabdomyosarcoma in children: epidemiologic study and identification of a familial cancer syndrome. J Natl Cancer Inst 1969;43:1365–73.
264. Malkin D, Li FP, Strong LC, et al. Germ line p53 mutations in a familial syndrome of breast cancer, sarcomas, and other neoplasms. Science 1990;250:1233–8.
265. Malkin D. p53 and the Li-Fraumeni syndrome. Cancer Genet Cytogenet 1993;66:83–92.
266. Easton D, Ford D, Peto J. Inherited susceptibility to breast cancer. Cancer Surv 1993;18:95–113.
267. Hisada M, Garber JE, Fung CY, Fraumeni JF Jr., Li FP. Multiple primary cancers in families with Li-Fraumeni syndrome. J Natl Cancer Inst 1998;90:606–11.
268. Lloyd KM II, Dennis M. Cowden's disease. A possible new symptom complex with multiple system involvement. Ann Intern Med 1963;58:136–42.
269. Li J, Yen C, Liaw D, et al. PTEN, a putative protein tyrosine phosphatase gene mutated in human brain, breast, and prostate cancer. Science 1997;275:1943–7.
270. Steck PA, Pershouse MA, Jasser SA, et al. Identification of a candidate tumour suppressor gene, MMAC1, at chromosome 10q23.3 that is mutated in multiple advanced cancers. Nat Genet 1997;15:356–62.
271. Li DM, Sun H. TEP1, encoded by a candidate tumor suppressor locus, is a novel protein tyrosine phosphatase regulated by transforming growth factor beta. Cancer Res 1997;57:2124–9.
272. Lopiccolo J, Ballas MS, Dennis PA. PTEN hamartomatous tumor syndromes (PHTS): rare syndromes with great relevance to common cancers and targeted drug development. Crit Rev Oncol Hematol 2007;63:203–14.
273. Longy M, Lacombe D. Cowden disease. Report of a family and review. Ann Genet 1996;39:35–42.
274. Schrager CA, Schneider D, Gruener AC, Tsou HC, Peacocke M. Clinical and pathological features of breast disease in Cowden's syndrome: an underrecognized syndrome with an increased risk of breast cancer. Hum Pathol 1998;29:47–53.
275. Hemminki A. The molecular basis and clinical aspects of Peutz-Jeghers syndrome. Cell Mol Life Sci 1999;55:735–50.
276. Jenne DE, Reimann H, Nezu J, et al. Peutz-Jeghers syndrome is caused by mutations in a novel serine threonine kinase. Nat Genet 1998;18:38–43.
277. Hearle N, Schumacher V, Menko FH, et al. Frequency and spectrum of cancers in the Peutz-Jeghers syndrome. Clin Cancer Res 2006;12:3209–15.
278. Swift M, Reitnauer PJ, Morrell D, Chase CL. Breast and other cancers in families with ataxia-telangiectasia. N Engl J Med 1987;316:1289–94.
279. Swift M, Morrell D, Massey RB, Chase CL. Incidence of cancer in 161 families affected by ataxia-telangiectasia. N Engl J Med 1991;325:1831–6.
280. Vorechovsky I, Luo L, Lindblom A, et al. ATM mutations in cancer families. Cancer Res 1996;56:4130–3.
281. FitzGerald MG, Bean JM, Hegde SR, et al. Heterozygous ATM mutations do not contribute to early onset of breast cancer. Nat Genet 1997;15:307–10.

282. Wooster R, Ford D, Mangion J, et al. Absence of linkage to the ataxia telangiectasia locus in familial breast cancer. Hum Genet 1993;92:91–4.
283. Athma P, Rappaport R, Swift M. Molecular genotyping shows that ataxia-telangiectasia heterozygotes are predisposed to breast cancer. Cancer Genet Cytogenet 1996;92:130–4.
284. Chen J, Birkholtz GG, Lindblom P, Rubio C, Lindblom A. The role of ataxia-telangiectasia heterozygotes in familial breast cancer. Cancer Res 1998;58:1376–9.
285. Easton DF. Cancer risks in A-T heterozygotes. Int J Radiat Biol 1994;66:S177–82.
286. Cortessis V, Ingles S, Millikan R, et al. Linkage analysis of DRD2, a marker linked to the ataxia-telangiectasia gene, in 64 families with premenopausal bilateral breast cancer. Cancer Res 1993;53:5083–6.
287. Nevanlinna H, Bartek J. The CHEK2 gene and inherited breast cancer susceptibility. Oncogene 2006;25:5912–9.
288. Bell DW, Kim SH, Godwin AK, et al. Genetic and functional analysis of CHEK2 (CHK2) variants in multiethnic cohorts. Int J Cancer 2007;121:2661–7.
289. Schmidt MK, Tollenaar RA, de Kemp SR, et al. Breast cancer survival and tumor characteristics in premenopausal women carrying the CHEK2*1100delC germline mutation. J Clin Oncol 2007;25:64–9.
290. Dannan GA, Porubek DJ, Nelson SD, Waxman DJ, Guengerich FP. 17 beta-estradiol 2- and 4-hydroxylation catalyzed by rat hepatic cytochrome P-450: roles of individual forms, inductive effects, developmental patterns, and alterations by gonadectomy and hormone replacement. Endocrinology 1986;118:1952–60.
291. Forrester LM, Hayes JD, Millis R, et al. Expression of glutathione S-transferases and cytochrome P450 in normal and tumor breast tissue. Carcinogenesis 1990;11:2163–70.
292. Rebbeck TR. Molecular epidemiology of the human glutathione S-transferase genotypes GSTM1 and GSTT1 in cancer susceptibility. Cancer Epidemiol Biomarkers Prev 1997;6:733–43.
293. Rebbeck TR, Rogatko A, Viana MA. Evaluation of genotype data in clinical risk assessment: methods and application to BRCA1, BRCA2, and N-acetyl transferase-2 genotypes in breast cancer. Genet Test 1997;1:157–64.
294. van 't Veer LJ, Dai H, van de Vijver MJ, et al. Expression profiling predicts outcome in breast cancer. Breast Cancer Res 2003;5:57–8.
295. Paik S, Tang G, Shak S, et al. Gene expression and benefit of chemotherapy in women with node-negative, estrogen receptor-positive breast cancer. J Clin Oncol 2006;24:3726–34.
296. Esteva FJ, Sahin AA, Cristofanilli M, et al. Prognostic role of a multigene reverse transcriptase-PCR assay in patients with node-negative breast cancer not receiving adjuvant systemic therapy. Clin Cancer Res 2005;11:3315–9.
297. Perou CM, Sorlie T, Eisen MB, et al. Molecular portraits of human breast tumours. Nature 2000;406:747–52.
298. Sorlie T, Perou CM, Tibshirani R, et al. Gene expression patterns of breast carcinomas distinguish tumor subclasses with clinical implications. Proc Natl Acad Sci U S A 2001;98:10869–74.
299. Sorlie T, Tibshirani R, Parker J, et al. Repeated observation of breast tumor subtypes in independent gene expression data sets. Proc Natl Acad Sci U S A 2003;100:8418–23.
300. Perreard L, Fan C, Quackenbush JF, et al. Classification and risk stratification of invasive breast carcinomas using a real-time quantitative RT-PCR assay. Breast Cancer Res 2006;8:R23.
301. Carey LA, Perou CM, Livasy CA, et al. Race, breast cancer subtypes, and survival in the Carolina Breast Cancer Study. JAMA 2006;295:2492–502.
302. Hu Z, Fan C, Oh DS, et al. The molecular portraits of breast tumors are conserved across microarray platforms. BMC Genomics 2006;7:96.
303. van 't Veer LJ, Dai H, van de Vijver MJ, et al. Gene expression profiling predicts clinical outcome of breast cancer. Nature 2002;415:530–6.
304. van de Vijver MJ, He YD, van't Veer LJ, et al. A gene-expression signature as a predictor of survival in breast cancer. N Engl J Med 2002;347:1999–2009.

305. Buyse M, Loi S, van't Veer L, et al. Validation and clinical utility of a 70-gene prognostic signature for women with node-negative breast cancer. J Natl Cancer Inst 2006;98:1183–92.
306. Morris SR, Carey LA. Gene expression profiling in breast cancer. Curr Opin Oncol 2007;19:547–51.
307. Paik S, Shak S, Tang G, et al. A multigene assay to predict recurrence of tamoxifen-treated, node-negative breast cancer. N Engl J Med 2004;351:2817–26.
308. Wessels LF, van Welsem T, Hart AA, van't Veer LJ, Reinders MJ, Nederlof PM. Molecular classification of breast carcinomas by comparative genomic hybridization: a specific somatic genetic profile for BRCA1 tumors. Cancer Res 2002;62:7110–7.
309. Jonsson G, Naylor TL, Vallon-Christersson J, et al. Distinct genomic profiles in hereditary breast tumors identified by array-based comparative genomic hybridization. Cancer Res 2005;65:7612–21.
310. Barcenas CH, Hosain GM, Arun B, Zong J, Zhou X, Chen J, Cortada JM, Mills GB, Tomlinson GE, Miller AR, Strong LC, Amos CI. Assessing BRCA carrier probabilities in extended families. J Clin Oncol. 2006 Jan 20;24(3):354–60.
311. Evans DG, Lalloo F, Wallace A, Rahman N. Update on the Manchester Scoring System for BRCA1 and BRCA2 testing. J Med Genet. 2005 Jul;42(7):e39.
312. Euhus DM. Understanding mathematical models for breast cancer risk assessment and counseling. Breast J. 2001 Jul-Aug;7(4):224–32.

Chapter 5
Gastrointestinal Polyposis Syndromes

William J. Harb

Introduction

The gastrointestinal polyposis syndromes (PS) are characterized by the development of multiple polyps, characteristically colorectal, but occasionally involving the small intestine and (less commonly) the stomach. PS may be characterized by the histologic type of polyps found, being either adenomatous, hamartomatous, or hyperplastic. Additionally, they may be characterized by the mode of inheritance, being either autosomal dominant or autosomal recessive. Changes in both these types of characterization have recently occurred. Until recently, it was thought that all polyposis syndromes were inherited in an autosomal-dominant fashion. However, the discovery of Mut Y homologue-associated polyposis (MAP), which is inherited in an autosomal-recessive fashion, changed this [1]. Additionally, the (relatively) recent addition of hyperplastic polyposis (HPP) was unique as this was the first type of PS involving hyperplastic polyps. The last several years have been a very active time, both with the addition of these new PS and further additions to our knowledge base about the known ones. This chapter will deal with the different PS and the management of each.

Familial Adenomatous Polyposis

Familial adenomatous polyposis (FAP, formerly known as familial polyposis coli or adenomatous polyposis coli) is the prototypical PS [2]. FAP is characterized by the development of hundreds to thousands of adenomatous polyps in the colon and has an incidence of approximately 1/10,000. It is inherited in an autosomal-dominant

W.J. Harb (✉)
Baptist Hospital, Nashville, TN, USA
and
Cumberland Surgical Associates, PLC 2011 Church St. Suite 703, Nashville, TN 37203, USA
e-mail: billharb@earthlink.net; billharb@yahoo.com

C.N. Ellis (ed.), *Inherited Cancer Syndromes: Current Clinical Management*,
DOI 10.1007/978-1-4419-6821-0_5, © Springer Science+Business Media, LLC 2011

manner; therefore, men and women are equally affected and the child of a parent with FAP has a 50% chance of inheriting the mutation. However, approximately 25–30% of cases of FAP are new cases (index cases or those involving a new mutation), whereas the remaining 70–75% are inherited from a parent. The penetrance of FAP approaches 100%, meaning that essentially all affected persons will develop CRC. Death ultimately will ensue unless prophylactic colectomy is performed [3].

Polyps develop early in life, with the median age of development of polyps being 16 years of age (range 5–38 years of age) [4]. In untreated patients, the mean age of diagnosis of CRC is 39 years and the mean life expectancy is 42 years [3]. As in normal colonic mucosa, there is a predominance for left-sided polyps which translates to an increased risk of left-sided colonic and rectal cancer in patients with FAP.

FAP is caused by a mutation in the tumor suppressor gene *APC* (adenomatous polyposis coli). This gene is located on the long arm of chromosome 5 (5q21) [5]. Each person carries two copies of the *APC* gene (one on each copy of chromosome 5). The person inherits one mutation in the gene from either parent and the second mutation is a somatic (acquired) mutation (Knudson's two-hit hypothesis) [6]. Adenomas are then initiated when the second copy, or wild-type allele, becomes inactivated somatically by mutation [7]. The mutation results in a premature stop codon that causes the production of a truncated protein in the majority of cases (>90%) [3]. The production of this truncated protein can be important in the types of genetic testing for FAP. The location of the mutation on the *APC* gene has been found to have clinical importance. Mutations in the *APC* gene which are nearer the 5′ end of the gene result in classic FAP, whereas mutations nearer the 3′ end of the gene result in attenuated FAP (AFAP) [8]. Classic FAP with hundreds of colonic polyps has been shown to most commonly result from mutations of the *APC* gene between codons 169 and 1393 [9]. Additionally, desmoid tumors are more common in patients with mutations between codons 1444 and 1578 [10] (see Fig. 5.1).

Extracolonic Manifestations of FAP

Extracolonic manifestations of FAP are commonly found in affected individuals. These include duodenal adenomas, small bowel polyps, gastric fundic gland polyps, osteomas, congenital hypertrophy of the retinal pigmented epithelium (CHRPE), desmoid tumors, dental abnormalities, epidermoid cysts, hepatoblastoma, adrenal hyperplasia and carcinoma, central nervous system (CNS) tumors, and papillary thyroid cancer [11]. Some of these will be detailed below.

Duodenal adenomas can be one of the more difficult conditions to treat in FAP. When followed over a prolonged period, almost all patients with FAP will develop duodenal adenomas. As with colonic adenomas, if left untreated, duodenal adenomas may develop into periampullary carcinoma. It has been shown that duodenal carcinoma is a common cause of death in patients with FAP [12]; in fact, duodenal carcinoma has been shown to be the most common cause of death in FAP patients who have undergone colectomy [13].

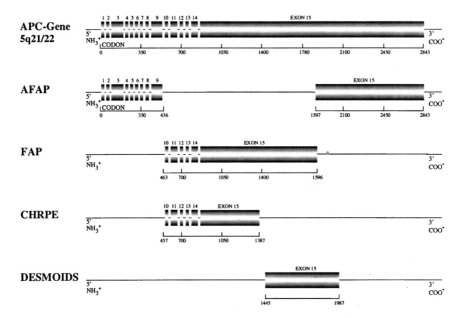

Fig. 5.1 Genotype/phenotype correlation of the APC gene. *FAP* familial adenomatous polyposis; *CHRPE* congenital hypertrophy of the retinal pigment epithelium. (From Hernegger et al. [8]. Reprinted with kind permission of Springer Science+Business Media.)

Duodenal adenomas are essentially universal in FAP. Groves performed upper endoscopy on 114 patients with FAP and found that 97% developed duodenal adenomas. Even those patients *without* adenomas developed adenomatous changes in grossly normal appearing mucosa, emphasizing the need for random biopsies [14–16]. Importantly, the incidence of duodenal cancer ranges between 1 and 6%. The median age of diagnosis of duodenal cancer is 47 years of age [11]. Spigelman et al. have devised a classification system for duodenal polyps. This is to assist with both surveillance and treatment recommendations and to predict which patients are at risk for progression from duodenal adenomas to carcinomas. In the Spigelman classification, points are assigned based on both the number and size of polyps, histological type, and degree of dysplasia (Table 5.1) [15].

Groves et al. have prospectively evaluated this classification in a series of 99 patients. Six of these 99 patients subsequently developed duodenal carcinoma. Segregating the patients with duodenal cancer by their initial Spigelman classification, four of six had Spigelman stage IV polyposis and one of six were each Spigelman stage II and III polyposis. No duodenal carcinoma developed in patients with Spigelman stage 0 or I polyposis [14]. As is the case for desmoids, genetic testing may be able to predict which patients have a higher risk of developing peri-ampullary carcinoma. Matsumoto et al. found that mutations in the *APC* gene before exon 9 resulted in a lower incidence of duodenal adenomas than did mutations after exon 10 [17]. However, the specific genetic defect which causes duodenal adenomas and carcinomas in patients with FAP has not (yet) been

Table 5.1 Spigelman classification of duodenal adenomas

Points	Polyp number	Polyp size (mm)	Histological type	Dysplasia
1	1–4	1–4	Tubular/ hyperplasia/ inflammation	Mild
2	5–20	5–10	Tubulovillous	Moderate
3	>20	>10	Villous	Severe

Stage 0, 0 points; stage I, 1–4 points; stage II, 5–6 points; stage III, 7–8 points; stage IV, 9–12 points
Source: Data from Spigelman [15]

identified. Further controversies in the management of duodenal adenomas in FAP include the type of surgical treatment indicated (duodenotomy with polypectomy vs. pancreaticoduodenectomy).

Although not as frequent as colonic or duodenal lesions, jejunoileal polyps (small bowel polyps) are still a common finding. Estimates of the prevalence of these are 50% for jejunal polyps and 20% for ileal polyps. The finding of small bowel carcinoma is uncommon in FAP, indicating the low malignant potential of jejunoileal polyps. As such, the role of screening for these in patients with FAP is not advocated [3]. However, with the increasing role of capsule endoscopy (and increasing accuracy as compared with contrast radiography), it may be that screening and/or surveillance of the small intestine in patients with FAP will increase in the future.

Gastric polyps are also commonly found in FAP. Histologic types of gastric polyps found in FAP include hyperplastic, hamartomatous, and adenomatous polyps. While fundic gland polyps are ubiquitous in patients with FAP, adenomatous polyps are less common and show a geographic variance, being more common in Japan [13].

Osteomas are the only extra-colonic manifestation in FAP which involve the skeletal system. The most common location is in the body of the mandible; however, they are also present in the skull as well as the long bones [13]. Osteomas occur with enough frequency that some had previously suggested screening for FAP by mandibular panorex X-ray. However, due to progress in medical technology, this is believed by most to be unnecessary. Additionally, while they were once thought to be very common (90%), recent studies have challenged this notion. A Cleveland Clinic study revealed that only 14% of 51 patients had significant lesions on re-review of X-rays [18].

Congenital hypertrophy of the retinal pigment epithelium (CHRPE) is another finding that has been thought to be almost universal in FAP. CHRPE is asymptomatic, and when bilateral, suggests that the patient should be evaluated for FAP [19]. As with X-rays (panorex) of the mandible to detect osteomas, some have suggested retinal exams to detect CHRPE as a screening modality for FAP. Data from the Cleveland Clinic indicate that approximately two-thirds of FAP families have four or more CHRPE lesions in both eyes [20]. Iwama noted that CHRPE was more common in patients with exostosis or desmoid tumors [21]. Morton et al. evaluated the utility of indirect opthalmoscopy in the detection of CHRPE. Seventy-five subjects from 25 families with FAP were evaluated. Using CHRPE as an indicator for FAP, the sensitivity was 84% and the specificity was 94% [22]. CHRPE most commonly occurs with mutations in the *APC* gene between codons 311 and 1444 [23] (see Fig. 5.1).

Desmoid tumors are a source of significant morbidity and mortality in patients with FAP. Desmoid tumors are histologically benign, nonmetastasizing fibrous tumors. The location of desmoids in patients with FAP include extra-abdominal, mesenteric, retroperitoneal, and incisional; most commonly they develop either intra-abdominally or in the surgical incision [24]. The main risk factors for desmoid tumors include previous surgery, female sex, family history, and *APC* mutation location. They represent the second most common cause of death after CRC [25], and are more common in females with a female:male ratio of 1.5:1. Additionally, most develop during the third decade of life [26]. However, it should be noted that the biggest risk factor is previous abdominal surgery. In fact, the finding of a desmoid preoperatively is uncommon. Two different studies have demonstrated that the median time after colectomy to the diagnosis of desmoids was 5 years [25, 26]. The lifetime risk of desmoids in FAP is approximately 20% [26]; however, only 2% of all desmoid tumors are associated with FAP. A review from the Mayo Clinic revealed that 11 of 196 patients with FAP (5.6%) developed desmoid tumors. Although family history is a known risk factor for the development of desmoids, none of the patients in the Mayo series had a family history of desmoids. Seven of the 11 patients developed mesenteric desmoids, while the remaining four developed abdominal wall desmoids. Church et al. have developed a staging system whereby desmoid tumors are staged I–IV [27] (see Table 5.2).

Dental abnormalities associated with FAP include impacted and supernumerary teeth, compound odontomas, and abnormal root formation [28–31]. As in other extra-colonic manifestations of FAP, the location of the *APC* mutation has also been applied to dental abnormalities. Oku et al. identified five members in a single family who had dental dysplasia and multiple osteomas of the mandible. Mutational analysis identified a one-base deletion at codon 1556 [32].

Skin findings are also part of the spectrum of FAP. These include epidermoid cysts (sebaceous cysts) and pilomatrixomas. One large series examining cutaneous manifestations of FAP was by Leppard and Bussey in 1975. They examined 196

Table 5.2 Staging of desmoid tumors

I	Asymptomatic, small, found incidentally	Observation/NSAIDs
II	Symptomatic, not growing, <10 cm	Tamoxifen/Raloxifene + NSAID Resection if feasible
III	Symptomatic and 11–20 cm or asymptomatic and slowly growing	Resection if feasible Tamoxifen/Raloxifene + NSAID Addition of chemotherapy
IV	Symptomatic and >20 cm or rapid growth	Resection if feasible Chemotherapy/radiation

Source: Data from Church et al. [27]

members of 15 families with Gardner's syndrome. Thirty-nine of 74 patients (53%) had epidermoid cysts. Importantly, they noted that these often developed prior to the onset of colorectal polyps. Although this work is over 30 years old, it is important to note their conclusion that the presence of epidermoid cysts in children should be an indication for sigmoidoscopy once the child reaches 14 years of age, even in the absence of a family history of FAP [33].

Pilomatrixomas are another cutaneous finding present in Gardner's syndrome. Eponymously known as the calcifying epithelioma of Malherbe, it is a benign tumor of the skin most commonly found in the head and neck that is derived from the hair follicle [34].

FAP also includes several variants. It is now recognized that the location of the mutation in the *APC* gene governs the phenotypic manifestations. Therefore, these variants, such as Gardner's syndrome and Turcot's syndrome, are now included within FAP. Gardner's syndrome includes FAP with prominent extra-intestinal manifestations. These have been discussed previously (see the specific extra-intestinal manifestations described above) and include osteomas, CHRPE, epidermoid cysts, dental abnormalities, and desmoid tumors. Additionally, Turcot's syndrome (TS) is the association of FAP and CNS tumors. It was first described in 1949 [35]. CNS tumors associated with TS typically include medulloblastomas and glioblastomas. Paraf et al. divided patients with CNS tumors into two groups: Those with glioblastomas and colorectal adenomas (called brain tumor-polyposis or BTP type I), and those with medulloblastomas and FAP (BTP type II). They noted that most glioblastomas occurred prior to age 20, thus suggesting a genetic link, possibly hereditary nonpolyposis colorectal cancer (HNPCC, also known as Lynch syndrome), since most of these patients were found to have germline mutations in the mismatch repair genes [36].

Genetic Testing for FAP

Several years ago, the prevailing thought was that FAP was a clinical diagnosis, being diagnosed whenever a patient was found to have more than 100 colorectal adenomas. However, the discovery of MAP and AFAP has changed that. First was the discovery of AFAP, which is clinically different in that fewer polyps are present. Additionally, polyps and colorectal cancer develop at a later age in AFAP. Second, MAP (see below) is a recently discovered syndrome which includes patients who clinically have numerous polyps, but do not have an *APC* gene mutation. A significant proportion of these patients have been found to have a mutation in the *MYH* gene (Mut Y homologue), which is inherited in an autosomal-recessive fashion. Therefore, genetic testing is required to determine which PS is present. For the proband, this can begin either with a protein truncation test (PTT) or germline analysis. As noted previously, persons with *APC* gene mutations produce *APC* genes which are shorter than normal (truncated); therefore the PTT will determine whether the *APC* gene is of normal size. Miyoshi et al. found that 92% of patients with *APC* gene mutations produced a truncated protein [37].

If the PTT reveals a truncated protein or if clinical suspicion is high and the PTT is normal, the next step in testing is germline testing (sequencing of the *APC* gene on chromosome 5). Sequencing is the direct evaluation of the *APC* gene using DNA sequencing technology. This has been shown to identify the actual mutation in 87% of patients with FAP [38]. Additionally, for a relative of a patient with a known mutation, gene sequencing and site-specific analysis can be done to identify if the known mutation is present in that person (accuracy approaches 100%) [39]. Once a diagnosis of FAP is entertained and, importantly, prior to the initiation of genetic testing, the patient should be appropriately counseled regarding the implications of the test, whether positive or negative. This may involve the use of a certified genetic counselor. Obviously, a positive result will have a lifelong implication, not only for the risk of colorectal cancer but also for additional cancers. The patient should be aware that a negative result could be a false-negative one. Additionally, patients may also have concerns that a positive test result could lead to difficulties in obtaining or maintaining health insurance. Laws are now in place which should hopefully prevent the discrimination of patients based on a positive test result. More than half of the states have laws in place that restrict or prohibit the usage of genetic information when issuing health insurance [40]. In fact, Hall et al. could find essentially no well-documented incidences of discrimination by insurers based on results of genetic testing [41].

Another important issue is that of genetic testing in relatives of patients with FAP. As stated previously, if a person is known to have a defined mutation, testing for that specific mutation via site-specific gene analysis can be done in family members. If the result is a negative one, screening can be done as it would for the general population. A positive result should result in colectomy at an appropriate time, usually after the development of colorectal adenomas [42].

Management of FAP

Screening implies testing for a disease prior to the development of symptoms. Screening of the general population for FAP is not recommended due to the rarity of the disease. However, testing of relatives with FAP (children, most commonly) is indicated. For children of patients with FAP, testing should begin at puberty and involves flexible sigmoidoscopy until the time when adenomas are detected. At that time, full colonoscopy is indicated [3]. Colonoscopy is also indicated in first-degree relatives of patients of FAP at the time of diagnosis (if he/she has reached puberty). Screening for extra-intestinal malignancies associated with FAP is based on reviews of series rather than population-based data due to the rarity of FAP. Screening for thyroid cancer, as well as jejunal and ileal polyps is not recommended [11]. Screening for duodenal adenomas should begin at age 30, with follow-up exams dictated by the Spigelman stage of the initial endoscopy [11, 14] (see Table 5.1).

Attention has been focused on the use of nonsteroidal anti-inflammatory drugs (NSAIDs) for the treatment of polyps associated with FAP for a number of years now. The first report regarding the use of sulindac for regression of polyps was in

1983 and the first controlled trial usage was published in 1993 [43]. Additional trials were done using Celecoxib (a COX-2 inhibitor) instead of sulindac. Steinbach et al. randomized 77 patients with FAP to placebo or treatment with Celecoxib (either 100 or 400 mg twice daily) for 6 months. Baseline endoscopic videos were compared with follow-up endoscopic videos. A panel of endoscopists viewing the videos confirmed a statistically significant decrease in the polyp burden (defined as the sum of polyp diameters) and polyp number in comparison with both placebo and the 100 mg twice daily Celecoxib regimen [44]. Subsequently, Celecoxib was approved by the Federal Drug Administration (FDA) for the treatment of polyps in patients with FAP. A recent Cochrane review demonstrated that NSAIDs are associated with a statistically significant incidence of regression, but not elimination of polyps in patients with FAP [45]. However, recently identified problems with cardiovascular side effects of COX-2 inhibitors may call this into question.

Surgery for FAP

Colectomy for most patients with familial polyposis is indicated at the time of clinical diagnosis. Penetrance of the gene is virtually 100%, meaning that essentially all patients will develop colorectal cancer, with the median age of development of polyps and cancer being 16 and 39 years, respectively. For the following discussion, two terms need to be understood. First, total abdominal colectomy involves removal of the entire colon (cecum, ascending, transverse, descending, and sigmoid colon). Second, total proctocolectomy involves removal of the entire colon, as well as the rectum. Surgery for FAP always involves total colectomy; therefore the main surgical issue involving the treatment of FAP involves preservation or resection of the rectum. As such, the surgical options for FAP include total abdominal colectomy with ileorectal anastomosis (TAC/IRA), total proctocolectomy with ileal pouch–anal anastomosis (TPC/IPAA), and total proctocolectomy with ileostomy (TPC/I). After the development of the ileal pouch–anal anastomosis by Parks and Nicholls in 1978 [46], the use of TPC/I declined in use. Several reasons for its current use include: (1) the patient with a distal rectal cancer in whom an oncologic resection cannot be done with preservation of the sphincter complex; (2) a patient who is unwilling to accept possible consequences of ileal pouch construction, such as multiple bowel movements daily or sexual side-effects; and (3) a patient who has fecal incontinence (although an uncommon indication in the age group who undergo surgery for FAP). It must be remembered that while TPC/I has declined in usage, many people are very happy with a well-done stoma. One final surgical option that is uncommonly used and will not be discussed here is total proctocolectomy with creation of a Kock pouch [47].

   In many minds, the optimal procedure for the treatment of FAP is total abdominal colectomy with ileorectal anastomosis (TAC/IRA). Preservation of the rectum (i.e., total abdominal colectomy) is preferred for several reasons. First, TPC is associated with known risks of pelvic surgery, such as sexual and bladder dysfunction and impaired fertility. Preservation of the rectum avoids the pelvic dissection necessary with proctectomy (removal of the rectum). While the incidence of these risks inherent in pelvic surgery is lower when the resection is done for benign disease (such as FAP in the absence of rectal cancer) than when proctectomy is done for malignancy, this risk is still present. In males, damage to the pelvic sympathetic and parasympathetic nerves results in retrograde ejaculation and impotence, respectively. The reported incidence is 2–6% [48]. Sexual side-effects in females are more common and include vaginal dryness and dyspareunia. The reported incidence of these has been as high as 25–35% [48, 49]. Secondly, continence is better when the rectum is preserved due to the normal function of the rectum as a fecal reservoir. Therefore, the functional outcome in patients undergoing TAC/IRA is slightly better than that in patients undergoing TPC/IPAA. While the number of daytime stools is similar (4 vs. 3), there is a higher incidence of nocturnal leakage in patients who undergo TPC/IPAA (26% vs. 13%) [50]. Finally, TAC/IRA can be completed in a single stage, without the need for a second operation (closure of the ileostomy in patients undergoing TPC/IPAA).

However, all potential functional benefits obtained from preservation of the rectum must be weighed against the potential for development of rectal carcinoma. Multiple institutions have evaluated the risk of development of rectal carcinoma after surgery for FAP in which the rectum is preserved [51–57]. Table 5.3 summarizes these studies. In general, the risk of rectal carcinoma increases with age, length of time since surgery, and the number of rectal polyps present prior to surgery. A single polyp >3 cm is also a predictor of a higher risk of rectal carcinoma [58]. It must be recalled that even in patients undergoing surveillance of the remaining rectum, rectal cancer is not always detected at an early stage; some patients will have already developed either lymph node metastasis or distant metastasis. Therefore, the 5-year survival following the development of rectal cancer in patients who have already undergone total colectomy with ileorectal anastomosis ranges from 60 to 78% [56, 59–60]. For this reason, in patients who have undergone surgery with preservation of the rectum, endoscopic surveillance of the remaining rectum should be done every 6 months. All polyps >5 mm in size should be

Table 5.3 The cumulative risk of developing rectal cancer following an ileorectal anastomosis for treatment of FAP

Center	Year	No. of patients	5 years (%)	10 years (%)	15 years (%)	20 years (%)	25 years (%)	40 years (%)
Mayo Clinic [51]	1980	143	5	14	19	32		
St Mark's [52]	1985	174					13	
Cleveland Clinic [53]	1987	133		4		12		
Scandinavian Study [54]	1992	294	3.1	4.5	5.7	9.4	13.1	
Japanese Registry [55]	1994	322	4.0	12.8	24.2			
Denmark, Holland Finland, and Sweden [56]	2000	659		4				32
NCI in Milan [57]	2000	371		7.7	13.1	23.0		

Source: Table 4.3 reprinted from Merg et al. [11], with permission from Elsevier

removed [42]. In patients with FAP who are undergoing surveillance of the rectal stump, changes occur with the obligatory polypectomies that make the diagnosis of rectal cancer a more difficult one to make than in a patient without FAP. The rectum becomes scarred and the carcinoma may be more difficult to detect [61].

A patient who is unable to undergo surveillance or one whom is unwilling to comply with surveillance should make the surgeon hesitant to preserve the rectum and consider TPC/I or TPC/IPAA.

Although surveillance for patients who undergo TPC/IPAA is less frequent than for patients who undergo TAC/IRA, there has been debate in the literature regarding the required frequency of endoscopy of the anal transition zone and pelvic pouch. The prevailing opinion is the ileal pouch and anal transition zone should be surveyed between every 2 and 5 years [42, 62]. The incidence of polyps developing in the ileal pouch after TPC/IPAA has been reported to be 42% after 7 years [63–65].

Cancer has been reported to develop after TPC/IPAA for FAP. Removal of both the colon and rectum does not completely obliterate the risk of carcinoma; it does make it extremely rare, though. Carcinoma has occurred in both the ileal pouch as well as outside of the pouch. A recent review reported 13 cases of adenocarcinoma that had developed after TPC/IPAA for FAP [66]. Cancer has been noted in both double-stapled anastomoses (DS), as well as cases in which a mucosectomy and hand-sewn colo-anal anastomosis (HS) was done. A retrospective review from the Mayo Clinic examined this issue. Of the 29 patients who underwent pouch excision, 17% of patients had residual rectal mucosa between the external sphincter and ileal pouch when examined histologically. The importance of this is that this residual rectal mucosa is not amenable to surveillance as it is outside of the lumen of the rectum [67]. Some have proposed that the DS technique (which avoids the mucosectomy) may not only be a technically easier procedure, but may make the residual anorectal mucosa amenable to surveillance. The issue of whether functional results are better after a DS or HS has not yet been settled. A recent meta-analysis of over 4,000 patients suggests that functional outcomes are equivalent [68].

Attenuated Familial Adenomatous Polyposis

AFAP (also known as attenuated adenomatous polyposis coli, or AAPC), is a less severe of FAP. AFAP was first described in 1985 by Muto when he coined the term "flat adenoma" [69]. Henry Lynch, in 1988, described a HNPCC family with flat adenomas and hypothesized that this was a HNPCC variant and possibly, a new syndrome [70]. Lynch et al. thus proposed the term "hereditary flat adenoma syndrome" [71]. Lynch et al. further concluded in 1995 that AFAP was a variant of FAP [72].

As an attenuated form of FAP, patients with AFAP commonly have <100 polyps, which is significantly less than the number of polyps found in patients with classic FAP. Other clinical differences from classic FAP include a predilection for carcinoma of the proximal colon, as well as the fact that the mean age of development of colorectal cancer is much older than in patients with classic FAP. In contrast to a mean age of development of CRC in FAP of 39 years, AFAP patients have a mean age of development of CRC of 56 years. The mean age of patients when polyps are found in AFAP is significantly older than in patients with FAP. One study found a mean age of 44 years [8] (as compared with 16 years of age in FAP). Clinically, AFAP is similar to MAP (see below) and genetic testing is required to differentiate between the two. However, one important difference between AFAP and MAP is that AFAP is inherited in an autosomal-dominant manner (similar to FAP), while MAP is inherited in an autosomal-recessive manner. Therefore, colon cancer will be seen in a more vertical manner in AFAP (parents and children), whereas in MAP colon cancer will be seen in a horizontal manner, if at all (siblings with colorectal cancer).

As in classic FAP, mutations in the *APC* gene are responsible for AFAP. Also, as in classic FAP, *APC* mutations in AFAP similarly result in premature stop codons. The genetic mutation responsible for AAPC is usually a mutation of the *APC* gene which extends past codon 158 [73].

Management of AFAP

Genetic testing, consisting of either a PTT or germline testing, should be done when AFAP is considered. If a known *APC* mutation is present in the family, site-specific germline testing should be done; a negative result essentially ensures that the person does not have AFAP. In a person at risk for AFAP due to family history or a known mutation, colonoscopy should be done at age 15 years, in order that a classic FAP is not missed. If this does not reveal polyps, subsequent colonoscopy should be done at age 20 years. If this is negative (and the person has a mutation), colonoscopy should be done every 2 years. Colonoscopy should be done annually in a person with polyps and a known mutation. Polyps that can be endoscopically resected should be. When polyps become too numerous and surgery is required, the best option is TAC/IRA, as rectal carcinoma is less common than with classic FAP. In a person at risk for AFAP due to family history, colonoscopy can be done as per an average-risk individual in the absence of a genetic mutation [8].

MYH Associated Polyposis

The study of polyposis syndromes was changed in 2002 by the discovery of *MYH* (Mut Y homologue)-associated polyposis (*MYH* polyposis or MAP) by Al-Tassan [1]. Prior to that, polyposis syndromes were thought to be inherited only in an autosomal-dominant fashion. MAP is the first polyposis syndrome known to be inherited in an autosomal-recessive manner. *MYH* is a base excision repair gene [74]. An error in the base excision repair gene such as this will lead to somatic transversions in genes such as *APC* or K-*ras*. A single mutation in the *MYH* gene (a monoallelic mutation) will lead to a carrier and a biallelic mutation will lead to the disease.

Thus, it would seem that in order for a person to have MAP, he must have a biallelic mutation in the *MYH* gene. However, some recent research does indicate that *MYH* carriers do have a higher incidence of colorectal cancer than the general population. Jenkins et al. found a risk of 2.9 times that of the general population for monoallelic carriers and a risk of 53 times that of the general population for biallelic carriers [75]. Others have noted similar findings [76], while some others have found that the risk of colorectal cancer in monoallelic mutation carriers approximates that of the general population [77]. Two mutations, Y165C and G382D, account for the majority of cases of MAP.

MAP presents in a manner similar to attenuated FAP in that patients normally have *up to 100 polyps*. The exact number is variable and has been reported to be as high as 266 polyps [74]. However, this is never in the range of thousands of polyps found in patients with classic FAP. One report of 25 patients with *MYH* mutations found a mean age of 50 years in those patients diagnosed with colorectal carcinoma [78]. Extracolonic manifestations such as congenital hypertrophy of the retinal pigment epithelium (CHRPE), osteomas, and duodenal polyps have been seen in patients with MAP. As MAP is inherited in an autosomal-recessive manner, a high clinical suspicion is *essential* to obtaining a diagnosis; most patients will not have a family history of vertical transmission and polyposis in contradistinction to AFAP. Indeed, several families have been noted to have family histories of siblings with CRC (but not parents), as would be consistent (horizontal transmission) [79].

Lefevre et al. reported a retrospective review of 433 patients operated on for polyposis. Thirty-one of 44 possible patients with polyposis who were *APC* mutation-negative underwent germline sequencing of the *MYH* gene. Six of 31 patients (19.3%) were found to have a biallelic *MYH* mutation. The median number of polyps in these patients was 60 (range 30–266). Importantly, no patient with <20 polyps was found to have a mutation in the *MYH* gene [74]. Others have reported a higher frequency of *MYH* mutations in *APC*-negative patients. Jo et al. examined the incidence of biallelic mutations in a series of patients who were *APC* mutation negative (all patients with more than 15 adenomatous polyps were tested). 15.6% of patients (seven patients) with more than 15 adenomatous polyps were found to have biallelic *MYH* mutations [80].

To reiterate, the key to the diagnosis of MAP is maintaining a high index of suspicion. Patients with multiple polyps should undergo germline testing for a mutation in the *APC* gene. If this is negative, testing should be done for *MYH* mutations. Risk of inheritance from an affected parent to a child is thought to be <1% due to the penetrance of the *MYH* gene in the general population. However, risk of a sibling having the same genetic mutation is 25% (due to the autosomal-recessive pattern). At this point in time, most believe that genetic testing is indicated for siblings, but not offspring [74].

As this entity was only recently described, treatment and surveillance options are still not fully developed. Due to the autosomal-recessive inheritance pattern, most patients will be found to have MAP after the development of colorectal carcinoma. Risk of metachronous carcinoma is not yet known due to the relative youth of the disease. Recommendations for prophylactic surgery are not yet finalized, as well. As such, recommendations for segmental colectomy vs. total abdominal colectomy have also not been established. However, it would seem appropriate for TAC/IRA to be the preferred surgical treatment if the diagnosis is known before surgery. Leite et al. [81] examined whether prophylactic colectomy was indicated in MAP. Of the 19 patients who were *APC* mutation-negative, 10 patients were found to have biallelic *MYH* mutations. Of those ten patients, four patients had node positive colorectal cancer and the tumors of seven patients penetrated through the wall of the colon (T3 tumors). They concluded that endoscopy was not sufficient for patients with biallelic *MYH* mutations and that prophylactic colectomy should be offered. This review does suffer from the fact that it is a retrospective one.

As time passes and we learn more about MAP, more recommendations regarding screening, surveillance, and surgery will undoubtedly come as our understanding of this disease increases. Due to the youth of MAP, surveillance endoscopy recommendations are not yet available. However, many would agree that surveillance colonoscopy on an annual or biennial basis after the diagnosis is made is a reasonable recommendation [3]. Additionally, yearly endoscopy after colectomy seems to be a reasonable recommendation taken from other PS.

Hyperplastic Polyposis

HPP is a (relatively) recently described entity through which persons are at risk for colorectal carcinoma through a different pathway than the traditional adenoma–carcinoma sequence. Critical to the understanding of this disease is not only the hyperplastic polyp (HP), but also the serrated adenoma (SA) and the sessile serrated adenoma (SSA). The HP, the most commonly found lesion in the colorectum, is usually distal in location and has little malignant potential [82]. However, this is not the culprit for colonic adenocarcinoma in patients with HPP. Instead, it is the serrated adenoma that is responsible for carcinoma in these instances. The SA is an adenoma which has a superficial architecture similar to the hyperplastic polyp, but does have the potential of malignant transformation. Additionally important is the SSA, which can be both large and proximal in location [83, 84]. It is thought that this is another pathway for the development of colorectal carcinoma, one in which the serrated adenoma transforms into adenocarcinoma of the colorectum. This has prompted some to suggest renaming the condition serrated adenomatous polyposis [85]. Also, some have suggested changing the name from HPP to sessile serrated adenomatosis to reflect the emphasis on this fact. This is not to be construed to mean multiple sessile serrated adenomas, as this has yet to be identified [86].

HPP typically presents in patients in their fifth to seventh decade of life [87]. The idea that HPP results in a predisposition to the development of colorectal cancer has been validated by several authors. In a retrospective review of 13 patients with HPP (patients with either 20 hyperplastic polyps or a single, 1 cm proximal hyperplastic polyp), Hyman found that seven developed colorectal cancer [88]. However, not all are in agreement with this [86].

Due to the relative infancy of HPP, definitions of the disease are scarce. Burt and Jass [89] have described a working definition of HPP which includes (1) at least five proximal hyperplastic polyps, two of which are >10 mm in diameter, or (2) any number of hyperplastic polyps proximal to the sigmoid colon in an individual with a first-degree relative with HPP, or (3) >20 hyperplastic polyps distributed throughout the colon. This definition has been adopted by other authors.

Currently, the mode of inheritance of HPP is unclear. Evidence exists that it may be inherited on a recessive basis [90]. However, there is also evidence that points to an autosomal-dominant mode of inheritance [91].

Much of the current literature regarding HPS is composed of case reports and series of several patients. The largest series includes 38 patients [90]. Chow et al., in a retrospective review, found that 19 of their 38 patients had a family history of colorectal cancer. SA's were identified in ten patients. Importantly, ten patients ultimately developed colorectal cancer, once again highlighting the importance of heightened surveillance in this group of patients.

As to the genetic mutation which leads to HPP, the association between CpG island methylator phenotype (CIMP) and mutations in the BRAF proto-oncogene has also been recognized [86]. Much more on this disease will undoubtedly follow in the years to come.

Peutz–Jeghers Syndrome

In 1921, Peutz first described the association of gastrointestinal polyps and mucosal hyperpigmentation [92]. Jeghers, in 1944, added additional patients to the cases previously described by Peutz [93]. Peutz–Jeghers syndrome (PJS) is a polyposis syndrome characterized by the development of hamartomatous polyps throughout the gastrointestinal tract along with characteristic mucocutaneous hyperpigmentation. The polyps may bleed causing anemia. Additionally, polyps may cause intussussception, leading to small bowel obstruction. The most easily recognizable aspect of the disease is the hyperpigmentation. This develops most commonly on the lips (95%), but also on the buccal mucosa (83%). In older patients in whom the diagnosis is being considered, one should be sure to look for the hyperpigmentation on the buccal mucosa, as that on the lips does tend to fade with age. Other locations for the skin changes include the digits, orally near the gingival and hard palate, as well as near the nose and eyelids [94].

Patients with PJS are at an increased risk for the development of cancers, both intestinal and extra-intestinal. Common malignancies and associated risks for their development include breast (54%), colon (39%), pancreatic (36%), gastric (29%), and ovarian cancer (21%) [9]. PJS is most commonly diagnosed in the third decade of life [95].

PJS is inherited in an autosomal-dominant fashion [96]. The genetic basis of PJ is a germline point mutation in the STK11 gene located on chromosome 19 (19p13.3). This gene encodes for a serine-threonine kinase which functions as a tumor suppressor gene. Mutations in this gene are found in approximately 70% of patients who have a family history of PJS, but only 20–30% of people who do not have such a family history [95].

Due to the frequency of associated malignancies associated with PJS, screening recommendations have been developed (see Table 5.4). Additionally,

Table 5.4 Screening recommendations for PJS

Site	Procedure	Onset (years)	Interval (years)
GI tract	Upper and lower endoscopy with	10	2
	small bowel follow-through	10	2
Breast	Breast examination, mammography	25	1
		25	2–3
Testicle	Testicular examination	10	1
Ovary	Pelvic examination	20	1
Uterus	Pelvic ultrasound	20	1
Pancreas	Endoscopic or abdominal ultrasound	30	1–2

Source: Data from Ellis [39]. Printed with kind permission of Springer Science+Business Media

screening (and surveillance) for GI polyps and their associated complications is indicated in patients known to have PJS. The utility and cost effectiveness of screening for pancreatic cancer in patients with PJS has recently been evaluated by the St. Marks group. Due to the rarity of the disease and the frequency of pancreatic cancer in patients with PJS, they do not feel screening is indicated [97].

Polyps in patients with PJS should be endoscopically removed when possible. For polyps that are not endoscopically resectable due to size or other technical considerations (small bowel polyps), operative intervention is the next step. Intestinal resection should be avoided due to the high incidence of re-operative procedures for recurrent polyps, the fact that most polyps regress by age of 30 years, and the risk of short-bowel syndrome [98–100]. Enterotomy with polypectomy, which may need to be combined with enteroscopy and intraoperative endoscopy, is the management of choice.

Juvenile Polyposis Syndrome

Juvenile Polyposis Syndrome (JPS) is characterized by the development of hamartomatous polyps in the intestinal tract. Importantly, the word "juvenile" in the name refers to the histologic type of polyps, not the age of onset. The most commonly used criteria for the diagnosis of JPS is the presence of five or more hamartomatous colorectal polyps, hamartomatous polyps in a patient with a family history of JPS, or proximal GI tract hamartomatous polyps [101]. Additionally, the presence of dysplasia in a patient with sporadic juvenile polyps should make one suspicious of the diagnosis of JPS [96]. It should be remembered that juvenile polyps (even more than one) are not uncommon in children without JPS.

Mutations in two genes, *BMPR1A* and *SMAD4*, have been identified in kindreds with JPS. However, mutations have not been identified in the majority of patients with JPS. Obviously, the possibility exists that other mutations which have not yet been detected may be responsible for JPS. Genetic testing of first-degree relatives is indicated in kindreds where a mutation has been identified. In a person who has a mutation, both esophagogastroduodenoscopy (EGD) and colonoscopy should be done at the beginning of the teenage years. If polyps are identified and can be endoscopically resected, then endoscopy should continue on an annual basis. In persons who do not have polyps, endoscopy should be done at least every 3 years. Consideration should be given to total abdominal colectomy in patients with nonendoscopically resectable colonic polyps [102].

PTEN Hamartoma Tumor Syndrome

Both Cowden's Syndrome (CS) and Bannayan–Riley–Ruvalcaba Syndrome (BRRS) involve mutations in the *PTEN* (phosphatase and tensin homologue) gene [3]. Along with Proteus Syndrome, the three have now been grouped into a new syndrome called *PTEN* hamartoma tumor syndrome (PHTS) [103]. All three of the diseases in this syndrome have a genetic mutation in the *PTEN* gene. Proteus Syndrome has not been associated with the development of intestinal polyps.

CS is an autosomal-dominant disorder characterized by the development of hamartomatous polyps which are not thought to be premalignant. Characteristic of Cowden's syndrome is the appearance of multiple verrucous lesions on the face and extremities. Associated malignancies include thyroid cancer, skin trichilemmomas, and breast cancer [3].

Although there is little information regarding the risk of colorectal cancer in CS, patients with CS are not thought to be at increased risk for colorectal cancer [103]. Current screening guidelines for patients with CS focus on the increased risk of breast, thyroid, and endometrial cancer.

BRRS unfortunately has no established diagnostic criteria. However, several features are included in the clinical picture of the disease, such as hamartomatous polyps of the gastrointestinal tract, multiple lipomas, developmental delay, hemangiomas, as well as pigmented macules on the glans penis [104].

The genetics of both CS and BRRS involves mutations in the *PTEN* gene. While PTEN mutations are not ubiquitous to both, it does seem that *PTEN* mutations are more common in CS (85%) than in BRRS (60%) [103]. There does also seem to be a difference in the portion of the gene in which the mutation is found, as in FAP. In CS, mutations seem to be more common in the promoter region, whereas in BRRS, deletions of all or part of the *PTEN* gene have been noted [105].

Conclusion

Polyposis syndrome can be characterized both by their manner of inheritance (autosomal dominant or autosomal recessive) or by the histologic type of polyps which are found (adenomatous, hamartomatous, or hyperplastic). With the increased knowledge of the mode of inheritance of many genetic diseases, there has also been an increased focus on genetic testing and its indications. As we learn more about the genetic mutations of polyposis syndromes, we undoubtedly will learn more about the appropriateness of genetic testing. There also will be an increasing emphasis on genetic testing. Getting the appropriate patients into the hands of the appropriate clinicians will hopefully be the outcome. While surgeons and genetic counselors undoubtedly need to be attuned to this important subject, many patients with polyposis syndromes (and inherited colorectal cancer, for that matter) will go undiagnosed unless gastroenterologists become more familiar with genetic testing. Certainly, it is the gastroenterologist who is on the front line and is usually the one who diagnoses colorectal cancer.

References

1. Al-Tassan N, Chmiel NH, Maynard J, et al. Inherited variants of MYH associated with somatic G:C T:A mutations in colo-rectal tumors. Nat Genet 2002;30:227–32.
2. Cripps WH. Two cases of disseminated polyps of the rectum. Trans Pathol Soc Long 1882;33:165–8.
3. Strate LL, Syngal S. Hereditary colorectal syndromes. Cancer Causes Control 2005;16:201–13.
4. Bulow S. Familial polyposis coli. Dan Med Bull 1987;34:1–15.
5. Bodmer WF, Bailey CJ, Bodmer J, et al. Localization of the gene for familial polyposis on chromosome 5. Nature 1987;328(6131):614–6.
6. Knudson AG Jr. Mutation and cancer: statistical study of retinoblastoma. Proc Natl Acad Sci U S A 1971;68(4):820–3.
7. Jass JR. What's new in hereditary colorectal cancer? Arch Pathol Lab Med 2005;129:1380–4.
8. Hernegger GS, Moore HG, Guillem JG. Attenuated familial adenomatous polyposis: an evolving and poorly understood entity. Dis Colon Rectum 2002;45:127–36.
9. Abdel-Rahman WM, Peltomäki P. Molecular basis and diagnostics of hereditary colorectal cancers. Ann Med 2004;36:379–88.
10. Soravia C, Berk T, McLeod RS, et al. Desmoid disease in patients with familial adenomatous polyposis. Dis Colon Rectum 2000;43:363–9.
11. Merg A, Lynch HT, Lynch JF, et al. Hereditary colon cancer – Part I. Curr Probl Surg 2005;42:195–255.
12. Bülow S, Björk J, Christensen IJ, et al. Duodenal adenomatosis in familial adenomatous polyposis. Gut 2004;53:381–6.
13. Alarcon FJ, Burke CA, Church JM, et al. Familial adenomatous polyposis: efficacy of endoscopic and surgical treatment for advanced duodenal adenomas. Dis Colon Rectum 1999;42:1533–6.
14. Groves CJ, Saunders BP, Spigelman AD, et al. Duodenal cancer in patients with familial adenomatous polyposis (FAP): results of a 10 year prospective study. Gut 2002;50:636–41.
15. Spigelman AD, Williams CB, Talbot IC, et al. Upper gastrointestinal cancer in patients with familial adenomatous polyposis. Lancet 1989;2:783–5.
16. Ranzi T, Castagnone D, Velio P, et al. Gastric and duodenal polyps in familial polyposis coli. Gut 1981;22:363–7.
17. Matsumoto T, Lida M, Kobori Y, et al. Genetic predisposition to clinical manifestations in familial adenomatous polyposis with special reference to duodenal lesions. Am J Gastroenterol 2002;97(1):180–5.
18. Woods RJ, Sarre RG, Ctercteko GC, et al. Occult radiologic changes in the skull and jaw in familial adenomatous polyposis coli. Dis Colon Rectum 1989;32:304.
19. Corman ML. Colon & Rectal Surgery, fifth edition. Philadelphia: Lippincott Williams & Wilkins, 2005.

20. Heyen F, Jagelman DG, Romania A, et al. Predictive value of congenital hypertrophy of the retinal pigment epithelium as a clinical marker for familial adenomatous polyposis. Dis Colon Rectum 1990;33:1003.

21. Olschwang S, Tiret A, Laurent-Puig P, et al. Restriction of ocular fundus lesions to a specific subgroup of APC mutations in adenomatous polyposis coli patients. Cell 1993;75(5):959–68.

22. Morton DG, Gibson J, Macdonald F, et al. Role of congenital hypertrophy of the retinal pigment epithelium in the predictive diagnosis of familial adenomatous polyposis. Br J Surg 1992;79:689.

23. Nieuwenhuis MH, Vasen HFA. Correlations between mutation site in APC and phenotype of familial adenomatous polyposis (FAP): a review of the literature. Crit Rev Oncol Hematol 2007;61(2):153–61.

24. Durno CA, Gallinger S. Genetic predisposition to colorectal cancer: new pieces in the pediatric puzzle. J Pediatr Gastroenterol Nutr 2006;43:5–15.

25. Sagar PM, Möslein G, Dozois RR. Management of desmoid tumors in patients after ileal pouch–anal anastomosis for familial adenomatous polyposis. Dis Colon Rectum 1998;41(11):1350–5; discussion 1355–6.

26. Soravia C, Bert T, McLeod RS, et al. Desmoid disease in patients with familial adenomatous polyposis. Dis Colon Rectum 2000;43(3):363–9.

27. Church J, Berk T, Boman BM, et al. Staging intra-abdominal desmoid tumors in familial adenomatous polyposis: a search for a uniform approach to a troubling disease. Dis Colon Rectum 2005;48:1528–34.

28. Ida M, Kline SN, Spatz SS. Gardner's syndrome (intestinal polyposis, osteomas, sebaceous cysts) and a new dental discovery. Oral Surg Oral Med Oral Pathol 1962;15:153–72.

29. Wolf J, Jarvinen JH, Hietanen J. Gardner's dento-maxillary stigmas in patients with familial adenomatosis coli. Br J Oral Maxillofac Surg 1986;24:410–6.

30. Sondergaard JO, Bulow S, Jarvinen H, et al. Dental anomalies in familial adenomatous polyposis coli. Acta Odontol Scand 1987;45:61–3.

31. Carl W, Herrera L. Dental and bone abnormalities in patients with familial polyposis coli. Semin Surg Oncol 1987;3:77–83.

32. Oku T, Takayama T, Sato Y, et al. A case of Gardner syndrome with a mutation at codon 1556 of APC: a suggested case of genotype-phenotype correlation in dental abnormality. Eur J Gastroenterol Hepatol 2004;16(1):101–5.

33. Leppard B, Bussey HJ. Epidermoid cysts, polyposis coli and Gardner's syndrome. Br J Surg 1975;62(5):387–93.

34. Pirouzmanesh A, Reinisch JF, Gonzalez-Gomez, et al. Pilomatrixoma: a review of 346 cases. Plast Reconstr Surg 2003;112(7):1784–9.

35. Crail HW. Multiple primary malignancies arising in the rectum, brain and thyroid: report of a case. U S Nav Med Bull 1949;49:123–8.

36. Paraf F, Jothy S, Van Meir EG. Brain tumor-polyposis syndrome: two genetic diseases? J Clin Oncol 1997;15:2744–58.

37. Miyoshi Y, Ando H, Nagase H, et al. Germ-line mutations of the *APC* gene in 53 familial adenomatous polyposis patients. Proc Natl Acad Sci U S A 1992;89:4452–56.

38. Giardello FM, Brensinger JD, Petersen G. American Gastroenterological Association technical review on hereditary colorectal cancer and genetic testing. Gastroenterology 2001;121:198–213.

39. Ellis CN. Polyposis Syndromes. In: Ellis CN, editor. Inherited Cancer Syndromes: Current Clinical Management. New York: Springer-Verlag, Inc, 2004:134–65.

40. Hall MA, Rich SS. Patients' fear of genetic discrimination by health insurers: the impact of legal protections. Genet Med, 2000;2(4):214–21.

41. Hall MA, Rich SS. Laws restricting health insurers' use of genetic information: impact on genetic discrimination. Am J Hum Genet 2000;66:293–307.

42. King JE, Dozois RR, Lindor NM, et al. Care of patients and their families with familial adenomatous polyposis. Mayo Clin Proc 2000;75:57–67.

43. Giardiello FM, Hamilton SR, Krush AJ, et al. Treatment of colonic and rectal adenomas with Sulindac in familial adenomatous polyposis. N Engl J Med 1993;328:1313–16.

44. Steinbach G, Lynch PM, Phillips RK, et al. The effect of celecoxib, a cylooxygenase-2 inhibitor, in familial adenomatous polyposis. N Engl J Med 2000;342(26):1946–52.
45. Asano TK, McLeod RS. Non steroidal anti-inflammatory drugs (NSAID) and Aspirin for prevention of colorectal adenomas and carcinomas. Cochrane Database Syst Rev 2004;(2):CD004079.
46. Parks AG, Nicholls RJ. Proctocolectomy with ileostomy for ulcerative colitis. Br Med J 1978;2(6130):85–8.
47. Lepistö AH, Järvinen HJ. Durability of Kock continent ileostomy. Dis Colon Rectum 2003;46:925–8.
48. Oresland T, Palmblad S, Ellstrom M, et al. Gynecological and sexual functions related to anatomical changes in the female pelvis after restorative proctocolectomy. Int J Colorect Dis 1994;9:77–81.
49. Bambrick M, Fazio VW, Hull TL, et al. Sexual function following restorative proctocolectomy in women. Dis Colon Rectum 1996;39:610–4.
50. Kartheuser AH, Parc R, Penna CP, et al. Ileal pouch–anal anastomosis as the first choice operation in patients with familial adenomatous polyposis: a ten-year experience. Surgery 1996;119:615–23.
51. Bess MA, Adson, MA, Elveback LR, et al. Rectal cancer following colectomy for polyposis. Arch Surg 1980;115:460–7.
52. Bussey HJ, Eyers AA, Ritchie SM, et al. The rectum in adenomatous polyposis: the St Mark's policy. Br J Surg 1985;72:S29–31.
53. Sarre RG, Jagelman DG, Beck GJ, et al. Colectomy with ileorectal anastomosis for familial adenomatous polyposis: the risk of rectal cancer. Surgery 1987;101:20–6.
54. De Cosse JJ, Bulow S, Neale K, et al. Rectal cancer risk in patients treated for familial adenomatous polyposis: the Leeds Castle Polyposis Group. Br J Surg 1992;79:1372–5
55. Iwama T, Mishima Y. Factors affecting the risk of rectal cancer following rectum-preserving surgery in patients with familial adenomatous polyposis. Dis Colon Rectum 1994;37:1024–6.
56. Bulow C, Vasen H, Jarvinen H, et al. Ileorectal anastomosis is appropriate for a subset of patients with familial adenomatous polyposis [see comment]. Gastroenterology 2000;119:1454–60.
57. Bertario L, Russo A, Radice P, et al. Genotype and phenotype factors as determinants for rectal stump cancer in patients with familial adenomatous polyposis. Hereditary Colorectal Tumors Registry. Ann Surg 2000;231:538–43.
58. Church JM, Burke C, McGannon E, et al. Predicting polyposis severity by proctoscopy: how reliable is it? Dis Colon Rectum 2001;44:1249–54.
59. Heiskanen I, Jarvinen HJ. Fate of the rectal stump after colectomy and ileorectal anastomosis for familial adenomatous polyposis. Int J Colorectal Dis 1997;12:9–13.
60. Vasen HF, van der Luijt RB, Slors JF, et al. Molecular genetic tests as a guide to surgical management of familial adenomatous polyposis [see comment]. Lancet 1996;348:433–5.
61. Phillips RKS, Clark SK. Polyposis Syndromes. In: Wolff BG, Fleshman JW, Beck DE, et al., editors. The ASCRS Textbook of Colon and Rectal Surgery. New York: Springer Science+Business Media, LLC, 2007:373–84.
62. Gray S, Artioli G, Olopade OL. Genetics in clinical cancer care: prophylactic surgery in inherited cancer syndromes. In: Devita VTJ, Hellman S, Rosenberg S, editors. Cancer Principles & Practice of Oncology. New York: Lippincott Williams & Williams Healthcare, 2004:1–20.
63. Wu JS, McGannon ES, Church JM. Incidence of neoplastic polyps in the ileal pouch of patients with familial adenomatous polyposis after restorative proctocolectomy. Dis Colon Rectum 1998;41:552–7.
64. Thompson-Fawcett MW, Marcus VA, Reston M, et al. Adenomatous polyps develop commonly in the ileal pouch of patients with familial adenomatous polyposis. Dis Colon Rectum 2001;44:347–53.
65. Parc YR, Olschwang, S, Desaint B, et al. Familial adenomatous polyposis: prevalence of adenomas after restorative proctocolectomy. Ann Surg 2001;233:360–4.

66. Campos FG, Habr-Gama A, Kiss DR, et al. Adenocarcinoma after ileoanal anastomosis for familial adenomatous polyposis: review of risk factors and current surveillance Apropos of a case. J Gastrointest Surg 2005;9:695–702.
67. O'Connell PR, Pemberton JH, Weiland LH, et al. Does rectal mucosa regenerate after ileoanal anastomosis? Dis Colon Rectum 1987;30(1):1–5.
68. Lovegrove RE, Constantinides MB, Heriot AG, et al. Comparison of hand-sewn versus stapled ileal pouch anastomosis (IPAA) following proctocolectomy: a meta-analysis of 4183 patients. Ann Surg 2006;244:18–26.
69. Muto T, Kamiya J, Sawada T, et al. Small flat adenoma of the large bowel with special reference to its clinicopathologic features. Dis Colon Rectum 1985;28(10):847–51.
70. Lynch HT, Smyrk T, Lanspa SJ, et al. Flat adenomas in colon cancer-prone kindred. J Natl Cancer Inst 1988;80:278–82.
71. Lynch HT, Smyrk TC, Lanspa SJ, et al. Phenotypic variation in colorectal adenoma/cancer expression in two families. Hereditary flat adenoma syndrome. Cancer 1990;66:909–15.
72. Lynch HT, Smyrk TC, Lanspa SJ, et al. Attenuated familial adenomatous polyposis (AFAP). A phenotypically and genotypically distinctive variant of FAP. Cancer 1995;76:2427–33.
73. Jass JR. What's new in hereditary colorectal cancer? Arch Pathol Lab Med 2005;129:1380–84.
74. Lefevre JH, Rodrique CM, Mourra N, et al. Implication of MYH in colorectal polyposis. Ann Surg 2006;244(6):874–9; discussion 879–80.
75. Jenkins MA, Croitoru ME, Monga N, et al. Risk of colorectal cancer in monoallelic carriers of *MYH* mutations: a population-based case-family study. Cancer Epidemiol Biomarkers Prev 2006;15(2):312–4.
76. Farrington SM, Tenesa A, Barnetson R, et al. Germline susceptibility to colorectal cancer due to base-excision repair gene defects. Am J Hum Genet 2005;77:112–9.
77. Olschwang S, Blanché H, de Moncuit C, et al. Similar colorectal cancer risk in patients with monoallelic and biallelic mutations in the MYH gene identified in a population with adenomatous polyposis. Genet Test 2007;11(3):315–20.
78. Sampson JR, Dolwani S, Jones S, et al. Autosomal recessive colorectal adenomatous polyposis due to inherited mutations of MYH. Lancet 2003;362(9377):39–41.
79. Bouguen G, Manfredi S, Blayau M, et al. Colorectal adenomatous polyposis associated with MYH mutations: genotype and phenotype characteristics. Dis Colon Rectum 2007;50(10):1612–7.
80. Jo WS, Bandipalliam P, Shannon KM, et al. Correlation of polyp number and family history of colon cancer with germline MYH mutations. Clin Gastroenterol Hepatol 2005;3(10):1022–8.
81. Leite JS, Isidro G, Martins M, et al. Is prophylactic colectomy indicated in patients with MYH-associated polyposis? Colorectal Dis 2005;7(4):327–31.
82. Day DW, Jass JR, Price AB, et al. Morson and Dawson's Gastrointestinal Pathology, fourth edition. Malden, MS: Blackwell Science, 2003.
83. Goldstein NS, Bhanot P, Odisth E, et al. Hyperplastic-like colon polyps that preceded microsatellite-unstable adenocarcinomas. Am J Clin Pathol 2003;119:778–96.
84. Torlakovic E, Skovlund E, Snover DC, et al. Morphologic reappraisal of serrated colorectal polyps. Am J Surg Pathol 2003;27:65–81.
85. Torlakovic E, Snover DC. Serrated adenomatous polyposis in humans. Gastroenterology 1996;110:748.
86. Young J, Jass JR. The case for a genetic predisposition to serrated neoplasia in the colorectum: hypothesis and review of the literature. Cancer Epidemiol Biomarkers Prev 2006;15(10):1778–84.
87. Snover DC, Jass JR, Fenoglio-Preiser C, et al. Serrated polyps of the large intestine: a morphologic and molecular review of an evolving concept. Am J Clin Pathol 2005;124:380–91.
88. Hyman NH, Anderson P, Blasyk H. Hyperplastic polyposis and the risk of colorectal cancer. Dis Colon Rectum 2004;47(12):2101–4.

89. Burt R, Jass JR. Hyperplastic Polyposis. In: Hamilton SR, Aaltonen LA, editors. Pathology and Genetics of Tumors of the Digestive System. Lyon: IARC Press, 2000:135–6.
90. Chow E, Lipton I, Lynch E, et al. Hyperplastic polyposis syndrome: phenotypic presentations and the role of MBD4 and MYH. Gastroenterology 2006;131:30–9.
91. Young J, Baarker MA, Simms LA, et al. Evidence for BRAF mutation and variable levels of microsatellite instability in a syndrome of familial colorectal cancer. Clin Gastroenterol Hepatol 2005;3:254–63.
92. Peutz JLA. Very remarkable case of familial polyposis of mucous membrane of intestinal tract and nasopharynx accompanied by peculiar pigmentation of skin and mucous membrane. Ned Maandschr Geneesk 1921;10:134–46.
93. Jeghers H. Pigmentation of the skin. N Engl J Med 1944;231:88–100.
94. Hood AB, Krush AJ. Clinical and dermatologic aspects of the hereditary intestinal polyposes. Dis Colon Rectum 1983;26(8):546–8.
95. Boardman LA, Couch FJ, Burgart LJ, et al. Genetic heterogeneity in Peutz–Jeghers syndrome. Hum Mutat 2000;16(1):23–30.
96. Attard TM, Young RJ. Diagnosis and management of gastrointestinal polyps: pediatric considerations. Gastroenterol Nurs 2006;29(1):16–22; quiz 23–4.
97. Latchford A, Greenhalf W, Vitone LJ, et al. Peutz–Jeghers syndrome and screening for pancreatic cancer. Br J Surg 2006;93(12):1446–55.
98. McGarrity TJ, Kulin HE, Zaino RJ. Peutz–Jeghers syndrome. Am J Gastroenterol 2000;95:596–604.
99. Spigelman AD, Arese P, Phillips RKS. Polyposis: the Peutz–Jeghers syndrome. J Surg 1995;82:1311–4.
100. Williams GT. Metaplastic Polyposis. In: Phillips RKS, Spigelman AD, Thompson JPS, editors. Familial Adenomatous Polyposis and Other Polypoid Syndromes. London: Edwards Arnold, 1994:174–87.
101. Jass JR, Williams CB, Bussey HJ, et al. Juvenile polyposis – a precancerous condition. Histopathology 1988;13(6):619–30.
102. Hunt S, Mutch MG. The genetic of other polyposis syndromes. Semin Colon Rectal Surg 2004;15:158–62.
103. Zbuk KM, Eng C. Hamartomatous polyposis syndromes. Nat Clin Pract Gastroenterol Hepatol 2007;4(9):492–502.
104. Gorlin RJ, Cohen MM Jr, Condon LM, et al. Bannayan–Riley–Ruvalcaba syndrome. Am J Med Genet 1992;44(3):307–14.
105. Zhou XP, Waite KA, Pilarski R, et al. Germline PTEN promoter mutations and deletions in Cowden/Bannayan–Riley–Ruvalcaba syndrome result in aberrant PTEN protein and dysregulation of the phosphoinositol-3-kinase/Akt pathway. Am J Hum Genet 2003;73(2):404–11.

Chapter 6
Familial Colorectal Cancer Type X

Deborah A. Nagle and Vitaliy Poylin

Introduction

Three to four percent of colon cancers occur in the setting of inherited or familial cancer syndrome. Currently approximately half of these are currently attributed to hereditary nonpolyposis colorectal cancer (HNPCC) [1, 2]. HNPCC is most commonly considered to be a familial aggregation of early onset, proximally based colon cancers, sometimes in association with other malignancies.

The field of inherited colon cancers was originally limited to familial adenomatous polyposis (FAP). Henry Lynch expanded the field with his description of a new heritable syndrome of colon cancer in the 1960s. His reports were based on observation of two familial clusters of colon cancers. Ultimately, two eponymous syndromes were described. Lynch syndrome type I is limited to families with heritable colon cancer only. Lynch syndrome type II includes families with extracolonic malignancies, most often endometrial and ovarian, as well as colon cancer [3]. Dr. Lynch himself introduced the term "hereditary nonpolyposis colon cancer" in 1985 to include both Lynch I and Lynch II syndromes [4]. Later Muir–Torre syndrome (multiple sebaceous neoplasms associated with visceral malignancy, most commonly colorectal cancer) was unified into the category of HNPCC due to similar patterns of inheritance and predisposition [5, 6].

HNPCC was best described as a syndrome with an autosomal dominant pattern of inheritance, early onset of colorectal cancer, and predisposition to colorectal cancers of the proximal colon. Additionally, multiple synchronous and metachronous colorectal malignancies in the absence of premonitory adenomatous lesions were noted. Cancers of certain extracolonic sites, most often endometrium and ovary, have a higher frequency of occurrence in affected patients [7].

Data collected from familial cancer registries soon provided evidence that HNPCC possessed a particular set of identifiable histologic features. These include poor differentiation, abundant mucin secretion, and marked lymphocytic infiltration

D.A. Nagle (✉)
Division of Colon and Rectal Surgery, Beth Israel Deaconess
Medical Center, Harvard University, Boston, MA 02215, USA
e-mail: dnagle@bidmc.harvard.edu

C.N. Ellis (ed.), *Inherited Cancer Syndromes: Current Clinical Management*,
DOI 10.1007/978-1-4419-6821-0_6, © Springer Science+Business Media, LLC 2011

[8]. Even though these features by themselves are not highly sensitive or specific, when combined with a positive family history, they are indicative of HNPCC. Improvement in molecular research techniques allowed genetic profiling of the affected families and a specific set of genetic mutations were identified. The most common cause of HNPCC was found to be a germline mutation in DNA mismatch repair (MMR) genes [9–11]. The MMR family of genes is tumor suppressor genes. MMR gene dysfunction is deleterious for microsatellite stability.

In an effort to standardize diagnostic, clinical, and research efforts, a strict set of inclusion parameters was proposed for hereditary colorectal cancer syndromes by the International Collaborative Group on HNPCC. The Amsterdam criteria, created in 1991, were based solely on family colon cancer pedigree and absence of polyposis syndromes [12]. These criteria were later revised in response to criticism that they were too stringent, in that patients with extracolonic manifestations of HNPCC were excluded from them [13].

The Amsterdam criteria address only clinical phenotypes. Among all the patients who meet Amsterdam criteria, only a small percentage will have the inherited genotype of germline mutation in mismatch repair genes. In effort to help determine which patients might benefit from genetic testing, the Bethesda criteria were developed. The first iteration (1997) and the Revised Bethesda Criteria (2002) combined pathological features of suspect colon cancers with extracolonic manifestations and Amsterdam criteria to identify those patients likely to benefit from genetic testing (Table 6.1) [7, 14]. Individuals who meet the Bethesda criteria should undergo diagnostic work up for specific germline mutations (defects in mismatch repair genes). If positive, these individuals and their relatives are considered high risk for early cancer development and require surveillance.

However, as familial cancer databases were expanded and more patients with hereditary colon cancer were identified, it became clear that there is a large subset of patients who satisfy the Amsterdam criteria, but do not exhibit the expected

Table 6.1 Amsterdam I and II and revised Bethesda criteria

Term	Criteria
Amsterdam I[a]	• Three first-degree relatives with CRC • Two generations affected • One family member below age 50 years • Excludes familial adenomatous polyposis
Amsterdam II[a]	• Amsterdam I • CRC cancer may be substituted by cancer of endometrium, small bowel or ureter
Bethesda (revised)[b]	• Multiple CRC or HNPCC-related cancers • CRC with MSI-related histology, <60 • CRC or HNPCC-related cancer in at least one first-degree relative <50 years • CRC or HNPCC-related cancer in at least two first and second-degree relative, any age

[a]All criteria must be met
[b]Any criteria can be met

HNPCC phenotype or have any of the expected genetic mutations [15]. In an effort to explain and categorize these patients, the term familial cancer syndrome X was described by Lindor et al. [15].

Clinical Evidence for Familial Colorectal Cancer Type X

Patients who satisfy Amsterdam criteria are expected to have early age of onset, but generally less aggressive, colorectal cancers when compared stage for stage with patients with sporadic colon cancers. Indirectly, they are also believed to have mutations in the MMR genes. However, a study by Wijnen et al. [16] examined 184 kindreds with familial clusters of colorectal or other HNPCC-associated cancer found that approximately 41% of families meeting strict Amsterdam criteria (I or II) did not have either genetic aberrations typical for HNPCC. The potential weakness of this study is that it examined only the most prevalent MMR mutations (MSH2 and MLH1). However, even though they did not examine all of the possible genetic mutations, the families studied were phenotypically different from typical HNPCC patients: they had significantly lower rate of extracolonic manifestations, and colorectal cancers they developed were more likely to be distal.

Subsequent studies by Lindor et al. [15] reviewed two disparate groups of patients among those satisfying Amsterdam criteria. Group A had identifiable MMR mutations by tumor testing, and group B did not. A total of 3,422 patients were examined. As expected, patients from group A showed a very high incidence of early onset malignancies. Patients from Group B showed a high rate of colorectal cancer in comparison to those with sporadic colorectal cancer. However, compared to Group A patients with MMR mutations they had a lower risk of colorectal cancer. More surprisingly, the risk of endometrial cancer (the most common extracolonic site in Lynch syndrome) was not higher in Group B patients than in the general population. Risk of malignancies at other sites, such as stomach, kidney, ovary, and small intestine was also lower than Lynch syndrome patients (Table 6.2). However, the risk of associated cancers was still slightly higher than those expected to be found in the general population.

Table 6.2 Standard incidence ratios comparing cancer risk in first- and second-degree relatives risks between families meeting Amsterdam I criteria with and without mismatch repair deficiency. Adopted from Lindor et al. [15]

Tumor site	MMR mutation	No MMR mutation	p
Colorectum	6.1	2.3	<0.001
Uterus	4.1	0.8	<0.001
Stomach	4.6	1.4	<0.008
Kidney	2.6	0.9	NS
Ovary	2.0	1.5	NS
Small intestine	7.6	1.6	NS

In a study by Mueller-Koch et al. [17], 41 families from familial cancer data-bases were divided into two groups, similar to Lindor's study. These authors showed that families without identifiable MMR mutations had significantly later age of onset of colorectal cancers. Families without documented MMR mutations developed colorectal cancers at a median age of 54 years vs. families with MMR mutations who had a median age of presentation of 42 years ($p < 0.001$). The study also found that colorectal malignancies in patients with proposed familial cancer syndrome X were also more likely to be in the distal colon when compared to patients with classic Lynch syndrome (79% vs. 32% of malignancies distal to splenic flexure). Synchronous or metachronous colonic lesions were significantly less common in the mutation negative group when compared to mutation positive group (1 vs. 12 patients, respectively, $p = 0.017$). For extracolonic tumors, this study also found a lower rate of endometrial cancer in the mutation negative group (5% MMR negative vs. 10% MMR positive). Finally, there were no synchronous or metachronous extracolonic tumors in MMR negative patients compared to MMR positive patients (17% with other tumors, $p < 0.001$).

These studies suggest that our current concept of HNPCC is limited by the definition that includes MMR mutations and resultant microsatellite instability. Another components of colon cancer development via mutation is the hypermethyla-tion pathway. Studies looking at early and right sided colon cancer identified the sessile serrated adenoma (SSA) pathway as a distinct cause of colon cancer. The SSA pathway is also caused by microsatellite instability.

The mutator phenotype pathway accounts for approximately 15% of all colon can-cers. It develops through mutations in MMR, primarily MSH2, MLH1, PMS2 and MSH6. This larger group includes Lynch syndrome (2-3%) as well as sporadic colon cancer cases (12-13%). Sporadic cases seem to develop in large part through the hypermethylation pathway (primarily BRAF mutation) are probably a significant component of what we are currently calling familial syndrome X. (Table 6.3).

Table 6.3 Comparison of Lynch syndrome and familial colorectal cancer type X with sporadic colorectal cancer

	Lynch syndrome	Syndrome X	Sporadic CRC
Age of onset	45	55	63
Location within the colon	Proximal	Distal	Distal
Multiple cancers	Common	Rare	Rare
Extracolonic manifestations	Yes	No	No
Genetic mutation	MMR genes	Unknown	APC
Mode of inheritance	Autosomal dominant	Probably autosomal dominant	Sporadic
Familial clusters	Yes	Yes	No
Pathological findings	Lymphocytic infiltration, abundant mucin	Unknown	Lymphocyte infiltration, mucin production uncommon

Screening and Surveillance of Patients with Familial Type X

The ultimate goal in describing and characterizing hereditary syndromes is timely diagnosis and appropriate care for patients. Effective care for individuals and families with Lynch syndrome involves informing and counseling affected, and at risk, subjects. Current guidelines for these patients include early and frequent colonoscopies: every 1–2 years starting at age 20–25 years. Endometrial biopsies and aspirations are also suggested for women with Lynch syndrome starting at age of 30–35 years; however, efficacy of this measure is controversial. Subtotal colectomy is the procedure of choice for Lynch syndrome patients who require any surgical resection of neoplasia. There is no firm data supporting prophylactic colectomies, either segmental or subtotal. Hysterectomy has been suggested for at risk individuals. In the setting of other planned abdominal surgery, prophylactic hysterectomy is supported. There is insufficient data for firm recommendations for prophylactic hysterectomy or oophorectomy [18–20].

These screening and surveillance guidelines used for Lynch syndrome patients may not be appropriate for familial cancer syndrome X patients, who show significantly different risks and age of onset of cancers.

How do we define familial cancer syndrome X (FCSX) patients? Those patients who meet Amsterdam I criteria and are MSI-stable or MSI-low are likely candidates for this diagnosis. Patients with extracolonic malignancies, i.e., Amsterdam II criteria patients, are not included. FCSX, by definition, does not evince microsatellite instability or germline mutations. If no established MMR defects are identified and Amsterdam I criteria are met, consideration can be given to classification of the patients as syndrome X.

These patients should be followed closely, although an optimal screening regimen is not yet defined. We propose the following, based on described clinical phenotyping (Box 6.1):

1. Amsterdam I criteria positive.
2. MSI-stable or MSI-low tissue typing.
3. No synchronous or metachronous extracolonic malignancies.

For surveillance of patients identified as FCSX, we propose the following schema:

1. A complete history and physical exam.
2. Genetic counseling and assessment.
3. Microsatellite instability testing (if not previously done).
4. Colonoscopy every 3 years beginning at age 40 years (or more frequently as directly by findings). Despite the left-sided predominance in these colon cancers, flexible sigmoidoscopy is not recommended. The variability, both practitioner-related and patient-related, in a sigmoidoscopic examination, precludes its effectiveness as a screening tool in this situation.
5. Routine gynecologic screening for women. At this time women with syndrome X do not have an indication for early endometrial or ovarian cancer screening. Screening recommendations for patients with sessile serrated adenoma/MSI

group of syndrome X are not clear. Since colon cancer in these pathways seem to develop relatively quickly, shorter followup periods are likely needed. If dysplasia is present, screening intervals should be short.

Conclusion and Recommendations

Our current diagnosis of syndrome X is a null diagnosis. In other words, confirming the absence of recognized mutations hinges on our ability to identify specific genetic alterations. This presents perhaps the biggest limitation and obstacle in characterizing this spectrum of disease. It is likely that we have not identified many of the possible mutations responsible for the clinical spectrum of inherited colorectal cancers. It is also possible that something as trivial as laboratory error may result in incorrectly classifying a patient into a less intensely followed group with potentially disastrous consequences. Finally, it is also possible that at least in some families, Amsterdam criteria are met by chance: MMR mutations can occur spontaneously and sporadically, and colorectal cancer is very prevalent in the general population.

Familial colorectal cancer type X describes a heterogenous population of those at increased risk of colorectal cancer. Undoubtedly our current definition includes some patients with sporacid MSI instability caused by hypermethylation. FCSX is currently differentiated from other inherited colorectal cancers by later age of onset, left-sided predominance of tumors and no identified genetic defect. It is distinctly different from Lynch syndrome and requires different follow up and treatment schedules. Since HNPCC fails to identify and accurately stratify these patients, some have called for the term to be retired and for these patients to be reclassified as having either Lynch syndrome or syndrome X colorectal cancer. This seems premature given our still expanding knowledge of colon and rectal cancer genetic pathways.

A great need still exists for further identification and characterization of this and other, another inherited syndromes. Now, with routine indentification of MSI instability by most clinical pathology departments, the proportion of patients previously described as having Syndrome X colon cancer will fall. As we continue our molecular exploration of affected families and new genes and mutation are discovered the FCSX category may be come even smaller. Environmental links may also be uncovered given the phenotypic similarities between these patients. Optimal surveillance regimes and inclusion criteria are evolving. For now, we should continue to identify and counsel these patients using Amsterdam criteria as guidelines, rather than dogma.

References

1. Brand, R.M., et al. Risk of colon cancer in hereditary non-polyposis colorectal cancer patients as predicted by fuzzy modeling: influence of smoking. World J Gastroenterol 2006. 12(28):4485–91.
2. Boland, C.R. Decoding hereditary colorectal cancer. N Engl J Med 2006. 354(26):2815–7.

3. Lynch, H.T., Lynch, P.M., Albano, W.A., Lynch, J.F. The cancer family syndrome: a status report. Dis Colon Rectum 1981. **24**:311–22.

4. Lynch, H.T., et al. Hereditary nonpolyposis colorectal cancer (Lynch syndromes I and II). II. Biomarker studies. Cancer 1985. **56**:939–51.

5. Muir, G.G., Bell, A.Y., Barlow, K.A. Multiple primary carcinomata of the colon, duodenum, and larynx associated with keratoacanthomata of the face. Br J Surg 1967. **54**:191–5.

6. Torre, D. Multiple sebaceous tumors. Arch Derm 1968. **98**:549–51.

7. Jass, J.R. Hereditary non-polyposis colorectal cancer: the rise and fall of a confusing term. World J Gastroenterol 2006. **12**(31):4943–50.

8. Jass, J.R., et al. Pathology of hereditary non-polyposis colorectal cancer. Anticancer Res 1994. **14**(4B):1631–4.

9. Sarroca, C., et al. Three new mutations in hereditary nonpolyposis colorectal cancer (Lynch syndrome II) in Uruguay. Cancer Genet Cytogenet 2003. **142**(1):13–20.

10. Wagner, A., et al. Molecular analysis of hereditary nonpolyposis colorectal cancer in the United States: high mutation detection rate among clinically selected families and characterization of an American founder genomic deletion of the MSH2 gene. Am J Hum Genet 2003. **72**(5):1088–100.

11. Wijnen, J., et al. MSH2 genomic deletions are a frequent cause of HNPCC. Nat Genet 1998. **20**(4):326–8.

12. Vasen, H.F., Mecklin, J.P., Khan, P.M., Lynch, H.T. The International Collaborative Group on Hereditary Non-Polyposis Colorectal Cancer (ICG-HNPCC). Dis Colon Rectum 1991. **34**:424–5.

13. Vasen, H.F., Watson, P., Mecklin, J.P., Lynch, H.T. New clinical criteria for hereditary nonpolyposis colorectal cancer (HNPCC, Lynch syndrome) proposed by the INternaltional Collaborative group on HNPCC. Gastroenterology 1999. **116**:1453–6.

14. Umar, A., et al. Revised Bethesda Guidelines for hereditary nonpolyposis colorectal cancer (Lynch syndrome) and microsatellite instability. J Natl Cancer Inst 2004. **96**(4):261–8.

15. Lindor, N.M., et al. Lower cancer incidence in Amsterdam-I criteria families without mismatch repair deficiency: familial colorectal cancer type X. JAMA 2005. **293**(16):1979–85.

16. Wijnen, J.T., et al. Clinical findings with implications for genetic testing in families with clustering of colorectal cancer. N Engl J Med 1998. **339**(8):511–8.

17. Mueller-Koch, Y., et al. Hereditary non-polyposis colorectal cancer: clinical and molecular evidence for a new entity of hereditary colorectal cancer. Gut 2005. **54**(12):1733–40.

18. Lindor, N.M., et al. Recommendations for the care of individuals with an inherited predisposition to Lynch syndrome: a systematic review. JAMA 2006. **296**(12):1507–17.

19. Smith, R.A. et al. American Cancer Society. American Cancer Society guidelines for the early detection of cancer. Cancer J Clin 2004. **54**:41–52.

20. National Comprehensive Cancer Network. National Comprehensive Cancer Network Practice Guidelines in Oncology, 2004.

Chapter 7
The Familial Atypical Multiple Mole Melanoma (FAMMM)-Pancreatic Carcinoma (PC) Syndrome

Adam I. Riker and Ramona Hagmaier

Primary cutaneous melanoma is the most lethal form of skin cancer if not detected and treated at an early stage. The incidence of melanoma continues to increase over the last decade, becoming the cancer with the highest rate of increase among Caucasians [1]. In the United States, the overall incidence of melanoma for the year 2007 is about 62,190 new cases, with over 10,000 individuals dying of metastatic disease each year [2]. It is estimated that 10–15% of all cases of cutaneous melanoma will occur in people with a hereditary predisposition for this disease, with most genetically based cases of melanoma closely linked to atypical nevi [3, 4]. The average lifetime risk for developing melanoma in the general population in the United States is about 1.5%; however, the same risk is markedly elevated in those individuals affected by a germline mutation within the CDKN2A gene, up to 76% over a lifetime [5, 6]. Additionally, carriers of such mutations have been shown to have at least a 13 to 22-fold increased risk for the development of pancreatic cancer [7]. Over the next few years, we will surely identify new mutations in this and other genes as well, which will enlighten us as to the complex genetic relationships between cancers of different histologies.

The first person to suggest that there may be a genetic predisposition for the development of melanoma was William Norris, who, in 1820, was one of the first physicians to describe a case of melanoma in the English literature [8]. He later published the first comprehensive study of melanoma, highlighting a series of eight cases of melanoma [9]. This manuscript is the first observational analysis of a group of patients with melanoma, accurately describing many of the epidemiological, clinical, and pathological features of patients with melanoma. Many of his observations remain true to the present day. Dr. Norris also performed, recorded and meticulously described an autopsy from a patient who died from disseminated melanoma, documenting such excerpts as, "the abdomen is filled with thousands and thousands of coal black spots…in endless profusion." It was also noted that the patient's father had also died of melanoma at a young age. In an 1857 article, Norris

A.I. Riker(✉)
Ochsner Cancer Institute, Department of Surgery, 1514 Jefferson, New Orleans, LA, USA
e-mail: ariker@ochsner.org

C.N. Ellis (ed.), *Inherited Cancer Syndromes: Current Clinical Management*,
DOI 10.1007/978-1-4419-6821-0_7, © Springer Science+Business Media, LLC 2011

stated that regarding melanosis, there was a "strong tendency to hereditary predisposition," further commenting that there was a strong correlation between the number of moles on a person's body and the development of melanoma [10, 11].

In 1952, Cawley et al. were one of the first groups in the modern era to describe an inherited predisposition to melanoma after noting a father with primary melanoma and his two children also developing melanoma at a young age [12]. In 1978, Wallace H. Clark, Jr., a pathologist at the Massachusetts General Hospital, had a passion for the morphology and biology of neoplastic pigment cells, becoming renowned for his descriptions of melanocytes and melanosomes seen with electron microscopy [13]. Clark described patients having melanoma as well as dysplastic nevi, and coined the term "BK mole syndrome," with the initials, "BK," derived from the name of a family afflicted with multiple moles and a predisposition to melanoma formation [14]. In 1969, he used the microscopic morphology of melanoma cells as a basis for classifying tumors into various stages of development. His studies revealed the progression of melanomas from a radial growth phase to that of a nodular or vertical growth phase. Clark also recognized variant patterns of the radial growth phase, further developing a classification system ("Clark's level"). He classified primary cutaneous melanoma samples based upon the extent of tumor invasion related to the anatomic layers of the skin, correlating the level of invasion to that of overall survival. This system constituted the first widely used prognostic model for melanoma [13].

In the literature, "dysplastic nevus syndrome," "familial atypical multiple mole melanoma (FAMMM)," "Clark's nevus syndrome," and "atypical mole syndrome" have all been used to describe a similar syndrome with the following components: a family history of melanoma in one or more 1st or 2nd-degree relatives, the presence of multiple melanocytic nevi, the presence of several atypical moles widely distributed over the skin, an increased frequency of multiple primary cutaneous melanomas, and a younger age at diagnosis [14]. Families with a hereditary predisposition for melanoma have been identified in populations on several different continents.

Due to a fraction of melanoma cases which could be attributed to an autosomal dominant mode of inheritance, researchers were led to investigate and analyze the genes implicated in inherited cutaneous melanoma. FAMMM is an autosomal dominant inherited disorder associated with germline mutations in the CDKN2A tumor-suppressor gene, which is located on chromosome 9p21. This particular gene encodes for two distinct proteins, $p14^{ARF}$ and $p16^{Ink4a}$, both low molecular weight proteins that have the capacity to block cell proliferation and are implicated in replicative senescence and tumor suppression [15]. Carriers of a germline mutation in the CDKN2A gene are predisposed to multiple melanomas and atypical nevi in addition to other malignancies. The $p16^{Ink4a}$ germline mutations have been found in approximately 20–40% of families from North America, Europe, and Australia that have a predisposition to melanoma, that is, having two or more 1st-degree relatives with confirmed cutaneous melanoma [16–18].

Further in-depth analysis of the CDKN2A gene has revealed that $p16^{Ink4a}$ is transcribed in alternate reading frames through alternate first exons [14]. $p16^{Ink4a}$ inhibits the activity of the enzyme cyclin-D1–cyclin dependent kinase 4 (CDK4) oncogene complex, subsequently catalyzing the phosphorylation of the retinoblastoma gene protein (RB1), releasing the transcription factor E2F-1 from the RB protein and inducing S-phase genes [14, 19, 20]. This, in turn, allows the tumor cell to progress through the early events in the cell cycle, specifically from G1 arrest through S phase. Since p16[Ink4a] binds to and inhibits CDK4, it prevents cell cycle progression, and these mutations that inactivate p16[Ink4a] prevent its inhibitory function on CDK4 leading to cell cycle progression and tumorigenesis [20, 21]. Others have identified p16[Ink4a] undergoing somatic deletion, mutation, or silencing in a number of neoplasms such as pancreatic cancer, glioma, and melanoma. Additionally, the CDK4 oncogene is located on chromosome 12q13. The CDK4 mutation is located at the p16[Ink4a] binding domain of CDK4. The p16[Ink4a] protein is unable to bind to CDK4 and thus, unable to inhibit the cyclin-CDK4 complex [1].

In 1993, it was Serrano et al. who first isolated the p16[Ink4a] protein, further demonstrating that the p16 protein binds to CDK4, thereby inhibiting the catalytic activity of the CDK4/cyclin D enzyme [22]. In the same year, Albino and Fountain suggested the involvement of chromosome 9 in the development of melanoma [4, 23]. The researchers analyzed melanoma tumors and cell lines by Southern blot analysis, showing that 86% of the samples had a loss of heterozygosity (LOH) at the 9p21 locus. This high rate of 9p21 LOH strongly suggested the location of a regional gene integral in the development of melanoma and ultimately helped researchers to further elucidate the exact role and function of the p16 protein. Nobori et al. subsequently identified the gene region on 9p21 which encoded the p16 protein by examining a panel of 46 cell lines including lung cancer, glioma, leukemia, and melanoma [24]. They discovered that a region proximal to the interferon gene cluster and the methyl-thioadenosine phosphorylase genes on 9p21 was homozygously deleted in 61% of the cases. They also found the presence of a germline mutation in the p16 sequence in a familial case of melanoma, thus solidifying the CDKN2A gene as having a major role in the susceptibility of individuals and families with germline mutations [24, 25].

In the literature, there is a wide range of findings regarding the worldwide incidence of CDKN2A mutations in patients with familial melanoma. Borg et al. analyzed affected family members from 52 families from southern Sweden, finding at least two cases of melanoma in 1st or 2nd-degree relatives within each family examined [25]. Polymerase chain reaction-single strand conformation polymorphism analysis was used to screen the entire CDKN2A coding region and the 5' portion of exon 2 for the CDK4 gene, with germline CDKN2A mutations found in 19% of the families and no mutations found in those families for the CDK4 gene. Nine separate families carried a 3 base pair duplication which resulted in the insertion of the amino acid arginine at codon 113 of p16[Ink4a], with one family having valine at position 115 replaced with glycine. Six of the families with the insertion of arginine at codon 113 had more than one family member with multiple melanomas. Thus, a total of 20 females and 11 males were affected by melanoma with the same six families found to have at least one family member developing pancreatic cancer, totaling nine cases overall. There were 2/9 family members with pancreatic cancer that also developed cutaneous melanoma.

Conversely, other researchers have challenged the generally accepted incidence of germline CDKN2A/p16 mutations in familial melanoma. Lukowsky et al. screened a small number of patients with either multiple primary melanomas ($N=40$) and familial melanoma ($N=15$), finding a novel mutation in the CDKN2A in only one patient with a multiple primary melanoma [26]. In support of this low incidence of germline CDKN2A/p16 mutations, Pjanova et al. examined 125 consecutive melanoma patients for such mutations, with no disease related mutations identified in any of the patients [27].

In addition to melanoma, other cancers have been observed in families with FAMMM syndrome. The second most frequently occurring neoplasm in patients with the FAMMM syndrome is pancreatic cancer [14]. Pancreatic ductal carcinoma is responsible for greater than 200,000 deaths worldwide, making it the 4th leading cause of cancer death [2]. It is an extremely aggressive tumor with an overall 5-year survival rate of less than 5%, the lowest 5-year survival rate of any cancer [2]. Mortality for this disease is almost at the level of its incidence. In the United States, it is estimated that 33,730 new cases of pancreatic cancer will be detected in 2007, with 32,300 deaths from the disease [2]. The mortality rate for pancreatic cancer is ~97%, with its poor prognosis primarily related to the late stage at the time of initial diagnosis, the lack of effective screening programs, and the fact that so few patients have surgically resectable tumors at the time of diagnosis. Approximately 50% of newly diagnosed patients will already have metastatic disease at the time of diagnosis, with most patients usually dying within 12 months of diagnosis [2, 18]. Smoking, chronic pancreatitis, diabetes, cystic fibrosis, high calorie diets, and certain occupational chemical exposures have all been known to lead to pancreatic cancer [28]. The most well-established environmental risk factor is cigarette smoking, estimated to account for 25% of all causes of pancreatic cancer [29]. Weight loss, painless jaundice, mid-abdominal pain which radiates to the back, and new-onset hyperglycemia or diabetes are the most common presenting symptoms of pancreatic cancer [18].

Studies over the past thirty years have estimated that anywhere from 4 to 16% of patients with pancreatic cancer describes another relative or family member as having this disease [29, 30]. Pancreatic cancer has been associated with ~25% of all FAMMM-associated families, with CDKN2A mutations identified in over 50% of such families with pancreatic cancer [31]. The joint occurrence of pancreatic cancer and melanoma has recently been given the name of melanoma-pancreatic cancer syndrome, also known as the familial atypical multiple mole melanoma-pancreatic carcinoma (FAMMM-PC) syndrome. The characteristics that distinguish familial cancer syndromes are multiple asynchronous or synchronous tumors, an inherited predisposition to one or more tumor types, and an early age of cancer onset [32].

In 1968, Dr. Henry T. Lynch was probably the first to describe a family with melanoma and multiple atypical nevi, consistent with FAMMM, in concert with pancreatic carcinoma [33]. This historical case series focuses on four families with extensive pedigrees that highlight the affected members with melanoma. Interestingly, in one of the four families, he documents the parents of the proband as not having melanoma, however the father having pancreatic cancer and the mother diagnosed with cervical cancer. Furthermore, two aunts were also found to have cancer, one pancreatic and the other with breast cancer. Melanoma was histologically confirmed in the proband, the proband's sister, and the proband's son. Thus, pancreatic cancer and melanoma was confirmed within five members of this single family over three generations.

Dr. Lynch continued this work in regards to genetically based cancer syndromes, publishing a study that convincingly showed that carcinoma of the pancreas was an integral cancer in the FAMMM syndrome [34]. Genetic analysis was performed on four kindreds with verification of FAMMM syndrome in over 80 affected family members in these families. Cancer at all anatomical sites revealed a 5-fold increased risk for FAMMM gene carriers, with an excess of carcinomas of the pancreas, lung, and breast [34]. He was also the first who proposed the syndrome that linked FAMMM to pancreatic carcinoma (FAMMM-PC) due to both cancers being identified as having mutations within the same gene, CDKN2A. In 1995, Whelen et al. identified a p16^{INK4a} germline mutation in a family with multiple cases of melanoma and pancreatic cancers, further identifying the same Gly93Trp mutation in all affected family members [32]. Goldstein et al. observed family members with the FAMMM syndrome and confirmed p16^{Ink4a} mutations had a lifetime risk of developing pancreatic cancer of 22 times higher than the general population [29, 35].

Vasen et al. performed mutation analysis in 27 families suspected of FAMMM, finding 19 families harboring a specific 19-base pair deletion in exon 2 of the p16 gene [36]. There were a total of 19 families inclusive of 656 relatives of which 86 members had melanoma, and, on average, families with the 19-base pair deletion exhibited 4.5 melanomas per family. The second most frequent cancer was pancreatic cancer, which was observed in 15 patients. Two families included four cases of pancreatic cancer, two families included two cases, and three families included one case each. The mean age of diagnosis of pancreatic cancer was 58 years. Based on their research, they estimated that 17% of carriers with a p16 gene mutation will develop pancreatic cancer by age 75, with a mean age at diagnosis of 58 years [36]. Interestingly, they did not identify any family member in suspected FAMMM families with pancreatic carcinoma unless they were found to have the p16 deletion in exon 2 [18, 36].

Bartsch et al. analyzed five families with at least one 1st degree relative with histologically confirmed melanoma and ductal adenocarcinoma of the pancreas. Several family members also had multiple dysplastic nevi. Genomic DNA of participating family members was isolated from frozen tumors and peripheral blood leukocytes. In 2/5 families with pancreatic cancer and melanoma, a truncated form of the p16^{Ink4a} gene was identified in the affected patients [37]. In one family, mutation analysis revealed a T-to-A base change at nucleotide position 324 which led to an amino acid change from valine to glutamate at codon 95. In another family, a G-to-A transversion at nucleotide 482 led to an amino acid change from alanine to threonine at codon 148. The median age of onset of pancreatic cancer was 55 years (range 45–67), and the median age of melanoma onset was 45 years (range 19–61). Even more recently, Rulyak et al. studied 370 members from eight families with multiple nevi, pancreatic carcinomas, and cutaneous melanomas [30]. At least one member in each family harbored a CDKN2A germline mutation, with 48.9% of the children affected with pancreatic carcinoma, melanoma, or multiple nevi compared with 16.7% of the offspring of unaffected parents. The work by Rulyak and colleagues represents one of the largest analyses of CDKN2A/FAMMM kindreds and provides further confirmation of the pancreatic carcinoma linkage to FAMMM.

In families with an increased genetic risk for developing melanoma, there has been no case of pancreatic cancer without an associated $p16^{INK4a}$ mutation [37]. To the contrary, pancreatic cancer has been observed in some of the families with this specific mutation. Explanations for this variation in gene expression include the influence of environmental factors such as nutrition, cigarette smoking, or the presence of modifying genes [36]. If pancreatic malignant conversion develops from a combination of multiple genetic events, examining multiple markers could lead to improved testing efficiency, especially in high risk groups such as chronic pancreatitis patients [38]. Over the past decade there has been significant progress toward understanding inherited susceptibility. Developments in molecular biology have enhanced the understanding as to the genetic aspects of cancers but much is still poorly understood. A review of the literature and a comparison of the different published reports analyzing CDKN2A mutations in FAMMM-PC is complex due to differences in the absolute criteria for FAMMM, differences in sample size, the different ways in which the probands are sampled, and the inability to tease out common exposures and environmental risk factors. In addition, much of the data on family occurrences of melanoma are obtained from interviews without subsequent verification as to the accuracy of the diagnosis.

Further research needs to examine other possible methods of identifying germline mutations both within coding and non-coding gene sequences. Since the CDKN2A gene is centrally involved with cell cycle regulation, further studies focused on germline alterations in other regulators of the cell cycle, such as CDK4, are needed. Additionally, we need to examine and clarify gene and environment interactions and how personal behaviors such as cigarette smoking and UV over-exposure may influence cancer risk. Discovering the genetic basis of FAMMM-PC could be of practical importance, quickly improving the way in which we educate the patient and family members as to their risk of developing cancer in the future. This, in turn, would lead to earlier detection of cancers and to developments of novel methods for diagnosis and treatment, such as the application of gene therapy for cancer treatment.

Multiple primary melanomas in a patient may signal a genetic susceptibility to melanoma in family members who may greatly benefit from thorough dermatologic screening beginning at a younger age, self-examinations, sun exposure avoidance, and other preventative measures. This also emphasizes the importance of obtaining a careful and thorough family history in all patients. Identifying patients with possible genetic links to an increased cancer risk is the key to providing prompt and appropriate surveillance programs for both the patient and family. This may reduce the mortality of cancer within these families. At least three studies reported the success of such surveillance programs, leading to the detection of melanoma at an early stage [1, 36]. For example, Puig et al. report that the molecular identification of CDKN2A mutation carriers resulted in the detection of eight early melanomas in their clinic that would normally not have been detected until a much later time [1].

The most important part of the clinical assessment and management of patients with FAMMM or FAMMM-PC syndrome will be to accurately document those individuals and families at risk. This entails a comprehensive history and physical examination, focusing on the family history, with the inclusion of a family pedigree if deemed necessary. In families with a strong history of melanoma, it is important to ask about other cancers in any other family member, such as breast cancer, osteosarcoma, soft tissue sarcoma, leukemia, brain cancer, adrenal cortical tumors (Li-Fraumeni), and pancreatic cancer (FAMMM-PC). It is important to ask about childhood cancers such as retinoblastoma, which in turn will result in much higher risk of developing other cancers (osteosarcoma, leukemia, lymphoma, lung cancer, bladder cancer) as an adult, especially melanoma (50-fold increased risk as an adult). Werner syndrome, xeroderma pigmentosum and ataxia-telangiectasis are rare genetic syndromes all associated with higher rates of melanoma and other cancers (stomach, breast, ovarian, uterine, lung, testicular) as an adult.

When assessing a patients risk and their family for developing melanoma or possibly one of the other genetic syndromes, spending some time to develop a thorough pedigree can be extremely useful in explaining the risks to the patient and family. For example, the risk of developing a primary melanoma in the general population is ~1%, however, for those individuals whom are found to carry the p16^{Ink4a} mutation, their risk is a markedly high 50% by the age of 50 and 76% risk by the age of 80 [39]. Furthermore, the risk of secondary melanomas is much higher in carriers, estimated that 15% of patients with multiple primary melanomas will be found to have a germline mutation in the CDKN2A gene, despite not having any family history of melanoma [16, 40]. The risk estimate for those patients with FAMMM and a known p16^{Ink4a} mutation for the development of pancreatic cancer is about 17% by the age of 75 years old [36].

Although there is no clear consensus on genetic testing for melanoma, one should consider genetic testing for germline p16^{Ink4a} mutations if two or more melanomas are identified within an individual or family, if a single melanoma and pancreatic cancer are identified in an individual or family, or if there are known relatives with the p16^{Ink4a} mutation. It is estimated that there is a <5% chance of individuals with two affected 1st-degree relatives of carrying the p16^{Ink4a} mutation, with this percentage rising quite dramatically to 20–40% for individuals with three or more affected relatives with melanoma. It is still somewhat controversial as to the overall benefits of genetic testing of patients for p16^{Ink4a} mutations, partially due to the known incomplete penetrance of this gene.

Therefore, it remains unclear exactly which patients will develop melanoma, pancreatic cancer or both in the future. A pooled analysis of CDKN2A penetrance showed a quite remarkable variation between different populations around the world, with a wide range of penetrance by age 50 for European populations (13%), and even higher for Australia (32%) and the United States (50%) [41]. Thus, the final decision for genetic testing of individuals for genetically-based melanoma, FAMMM or

FAMMM-PC syndrome will ultimately be made after a thorough discussion about the risks and benefits of the test between the patient and their treating physician. It is, of course, very helpful to have a professional genetic risk counselor who is well-versed in the various genetically inherited cancer syndromes; however, such expertise may not be readily available outside major universities or academic centers.

The Melaris® genetic test (Myriad Genetics, Inc.) is currently being offered to determine if a patient or any member of their family has a p16^{Ink4a} mutation, possibly indicating a genetic predisposition for the future development of melanoma and/or pancreatic cancer (www.myriad.com). It is currently able to screen for the known 50 unique germline mutations within the CDKN2A coding sequence, splicing region or promoter regions. It is important to clarify with all family members that if a single carrier is indeed identified with a p16^{Ink4a} mutation, it is incumbent that others are also tested in order to determine whether this mutation has been passed along in an autosomal dominant fashion.

There are several strategies that can be followed once it has been determined that an individual tests positive for the p16^{Ink4a} mutation. First, it is imperative that full and detailed discussion is completed with the patient, and of equal importance, with other family members. It is very important for the entire family to realize what their individual risk is, and often this will lead to further testing for possible p16^{Ink4a} mutations in non-tested family members. Secondly, the proband is treated according to current guidelines for the surgical management of melanoma, and once healed, should be given a detailed follow-up regimen consisting of close observation of all areas of the skin and thorough physical examinations. Although there are no standard guidelines for the continued surveillance and follow-up for patients with germline p16^{Ink4a} mutations, some general and sensible guidelines may be safely followed in most, if not all patients.

In terms of those patients being followed for the possible development of FAMMM-PC syndrome, we would recommend monthly, full body, naked skin exams by the spouse or significant other, followed by clinical examinations of all areas of the skin every 3–6 months for the rest of their lives. Although by far a consensus, a CT scan of the abdomen to exclude the interval development of a pancreatic mass may also be considered on a yearly basis. To exclude other possible genetically-based syndromes, such as Li-Fraumeni, we recommend monthly breast exams at home in addition to a yearly, bilateral screening mammogram beginning at the age of 35. Of course, we re-iterate the importance of minimizing exposure to UV-irradiation through the use of sun blocks, avoidance of tanning salons and prolonged exposure to the sun. The increased level of surveillance intuitively will lead to the earlier detection of primary cutaneous melanomas that can be biopsied for diagnosis and treated earlier in their course. This is also the case for the possible finding of a pancreatic mass that has developed very early in its course, thus making early surgical management much more successful.

In 2003, the American Society of Clinical Oncology updated their original 1996 consensus statement and policy on genetic testing for cancer susceptibility, setting forth specific recommendations related to such testing [42]. They clearly describe thew indications for genetic testing, focusing on the individual with a personal or family history suggestive of genetic cancer as those most in need of testing. Other topics discussed range from genetic counseling, special issues in children, confidentiality of familial risk and protection from insurance and employment discrimination based upon a clearly defined genetic predisposition to cancer. This policy statement was developed as a result of the efforts of the ASCO Working Group on Genetic Testing for Cancer Susceptibility, chaired by Dr. Kennith Offit, and offers a clearly written statement and recommended guidelines for an array of issues and problems that may arise as a result of genetic testing for cancer.

References

1. Puig S, Malvehy J, Bandenas C, et al. Role of the CDKN2A locus in patients with multiple primary melanomas. J Clin Oncol 2005;23:3043–51.
2. Jemal A, Siegel R, Ward E, et al. Cancer Statistics, 2006. CA Cancer J Clin 2006;56:106–30.
3. Goldstein A, Tucker M. Screening for CDKN2A mutations in hereditary melanoma. J Natl Cancer Inst 1997;89:676–7.
4. Haluska FG, Hodi FS. Molecular genetics of familial cutaneous melanoma. J Clin Oncol 1998;16:670–82.
5. Hansen CB, Wadge LM, Lowstuter K, et al. Clinical germline genetic testing for melanoma. Lancet Oncol 2004;5(5):314–9.
6. Somoano B, Niendorf KB, Tsao H. Hereditary cancer syndromes of the skin. Clin Dermatol 2005;23:85–106.
7. Rieder H, Bartsch DK. Familial pancreatic cancer. Fam Cancer 2004;3(1):69–74.
8. Norris W. Case of fungoid disease. Edinburgh Med Surg 1820;16:562.
9. Norris W. Eight cases of melanosis with pathological and therapeutical remarks on that disease. London, UK: Longman, Brown, Green, Longman and Roberts; 1857.
10. Balch CM, Milton GW. Cutaneous melanoma: clinical management and treatment results worldwide. Philadelphia: J.B. Lippincott; 1985.
11. Platz A, Ringborg U, Hansson J. Hereditary cutaneous melanoma. Cancer Biol 2000;10:319–26.
12. Cawley EP. Genetic aspects of malignant melanoma. AMA Arch Dermatol 1952;65:440–50.
13. Riker AI, D'Alessio M, Hagmaier R, et al. The surgical management of cutaneous melanoma. G Ital Dermatol Venereol 2007;142(2):171–95.
14. Czajkowski R, Placek W, Drewa G, et al. FAMMM Syndrome: pathogenesis and management. Dermatol Surg 2004;30:291–6.
15. Jones R, Ruas M, Gregory F, et al. A CDKN2A mutation in familial melanoma that abrogates binding of p16INK4a to CDK4 but not CDK6. Cancer Res 2007;67(19):9134–41.
16. Monzon J, Liu L, Brill H, et al. CDKN2A mutations in multiple primary melanomas. N Engl J Med 1998;338:879–87.
17. Goldstein AM, Struewing JP, Chidambaram A, et al. Genotype-phenotype relationships in U.S. melanoma-prone families with CDKN2A and CDK4 mutations. J Natl Cancer Inst 2000;92:1006–10.
18. Parker JF, Florell SR, Alexander A, et al. Pancreatic carcinoma surveillance in patients with familial melanoma. Arch Dermatol 2003;139:1019–25.
19. Sviderskaya E, Hill S, Evans-Whipp T, et al. p16Ink4a in melanocyte senescence and differentiation. J Natl Cancer Inst 2002;94:446–54.
20. Sviderskaya E, Gray-Schopfer V, Hill S, et al. p16/cyclin-dependent kinase inhibitor 2A deficiency in human melanocyte senescence, apoptosis, and immortalization: possible implications for melanoma progression. J Natl Cancer Inst 2003;95:723–32.
21. de Snoo FA, Kroon MW, Bergman W, et al. From sporadic atypical nevi to familial melanoma: risk analysis for melanoma in sporadic atypical nevus patients. J Am Acad Dermatol 2007;56(5):748–52.
22. Serrano M, Hannon GJ, Beach D. A new regulatory motif in cell-cycle control causing specific inhibition of cyclin D/CDK4. Nature 1993;366(6456):704–7.

23. Tsao H, Niendorf K. Genetic testing in hereditary melanoma. J Am Acad Dermatol 2004;51:803–8.
24. Nobori T, Miura K, Wu D, et al. Deletions of the cyclin-dependent kinase-4 inhibitor gene in multiple human cancers. Nature 1994;368:753–56.
25. Borg A, Sandberg T, Nilsson K, et al. High frequency of multiple melanomas and breast and pancreas carcinomas in CDKN2A mutation-positive melanoma families. J Natl Cancer Inst 2000;92:1260–6.
26. Lukowsky A, Schafer-Hesterberg G, Sterry W, et al. Germline CDKN2A/p16 mutations are rare in multiple primary and familial malignant melanoma in German patients. J Dermatol Sci in press.
27. Pjanova D, Engele L, Randerson-Moor J, et al. CDKN2A and CDK4 variants in Latvian melanoma patients: analysis of a clinic-based population. Melanoma Res 2007;17:185–91.
28. Jeong J, Park YN, Park JS, et al. Clinical significance of p16 protein expression loss and aberrant p53 protein expression in pancreatic cancer. Yonsei Med J 2005;46:519–25.
29. Klein AP, Hruban RH, Brune KA, et al. Familial pancreatic cancer. Cancer J 2001;7:266–73.
30. Rulyak SJ, Brentnall TA, Lynch HT, et al. Characterization of the neoplastic phenotype in the familial atypical multiple-mole melanoma-pancreatic carcinoma syndrome. Cancer 2003;98:798–804.
31. Habbe N, Langer P, Sina-Frey M, et al. Familial pancreatic cancer syndromes. Endocrinol Metab Clin N Am 2006;35:417–30.
32. Whelan AJ, Bartsch D, Goodfellow PJ. Brief Report: A familial syndrome of pancreatic cancer and melanoma with a mutation in the CDKN2 tumor-supressor gene. N Engl J Med 1995;333:975–7.
33. Lynch HT, Krush AJ. Heredity and malignant melanoma: implications for early cancer detection. Can Med Ass J 1968;99:17–21.
34. Lynch HT, Fusaro RM, Kimberling WJ, et al. Familial atypical multiple mole-melanoma (FAMMM) syndrome: segregation analysis. J Med Genet 1983;20:342–4.
35. Goldstein AM, Fraser MC, Struewing JP, et al. Increased risk of pancreatic cancer in melanoma-prone kindreds with p16INK4 mutations. N Engl J Med 1995;333:970–4.
36. Vasen H, Gruis N, Frants R, et al. Risk of developing pancreatic cancer in families with familial atypical multiple mole melanoma associated with a specific 19 deletion of p16. Int J Cancer 2000;87:809–11.
37. Bartsch DK, Sina-Frey M, Lang S, et al. CDKN2A germline mutations in familial pancreatic cancer. Ann Surg 2002;236:730–37.
38. Salek C, Benesova L, Zavoral M, et al. Evaluation of clinical relevance of examining K-ras, p16 and p53 mutations along with allelic losses at 9p and 18q in EUS-guided fine needle aspiration samples of patients with chronic pancreatitis and pancreatic cancer. World J Gastroenterol 2007;13:3714–20.
39. Bishop DT, Demenais F, Goldstein AM, et al. Geographical variation in the penetrance of CDKN2A mutations in melanoma. J Natl Cancer Inst 2002;94:894–903.
40. Hashemi J, Platz A, Ueno T, et al. CDKN2A germline mutations in individuals with multiple cutaneous melanomas. Cancer Res 2000;60:6864–7.
41. Goldstein AM, Chan M, Harland M, et al. High-risk melanoma susceptibility genes and pancreatic cancer, neural system tumors, and uveal melanoma across GenoMEL. Cancer Res 2006;66(20):9818–28.
42. Society of Clinical Oncology. Policy statement update: genetic testing for cancer susceptibility. J Clin Oncol 2003;21:2397–406.

Chapter 8
Desmoid Disease

James M. Church

Introduction

Desmoid disease is an overgrowth of fibrous tissue that presents in patients with Familial Adenomatous Polyposis (FAP) as a spectrum of lesions from flat, two-dimensional sheets to large, rapidly growing, three-dimensional tumors. FAP-related desmoid tumors can be confused with sporadic desmoids that occur in the general population with an incidence of two to three per million [1]. These sporadic desmoids are found in limbs and limb girdles, and around the spine. They rarely occur inside the abdomen, and when apparently sporadic intra-abdominal desmoids present, it is hard to exclude FAP even when the colon is normal. Perhaps the best way would be to examine the tumor for mutations in either *APC* or *CTNNB1*. All desmoid tumors have an overactive wnt/wingless signal transduction pathway with nuclear accumulation of B catenin but sporadic desmoids come to this differently from FAP-related desmoids. Sporadic desmoids over-express b catenin due to either an activating mutation in *CTNNB1* or a sporadic mutation of *APC* [2, 3]. FAP-associated desmoids have a germline mutation in *APC* [2–4]. Desmoid tumors, whether FAP-associated or sporadic, are a challenge because of their propensity to recur after surgery and the unpredictable effect of medical treatments [3, 5]. Desmoid disease in FAP differs from sporadic desmoid tumors in that it is largely intra-abdominal, usually follows major abdominal surgery, and is quite common in this particular subset of patients. Because of their site within the abdomen, FAP-associated desmoids can cause significant problems with bowel or ureteric obstruction, abscess, fistula, and symptomatic masses [6–8]. They are the third most common cause of death in FAP, after colorectal and periampullary cancer [9]. Resection is difficult as the tumors often involve the superior mesenteric artery, recurrence rate after surgery is at least 50%, and there is no uniformly effective drug treatment available [6–8].

J.M. Church (⊠)
Department of Colorectal Neoplasia, Sanford R. Weiss Center for Hereditary Colorectal Cancer, Cleveland Clinic Foundation, Cleveland, OH 44195, USA
e-mail: churchj@ccf.org

C.N. Ellis (ed.), *Inherited Cancer Syndromes: Current Clinical Management*,
DOI 10.1007/978-1-4419-6821-0_8, © Springer Science+Business Media, LLC 2011

Definition and Staging

Desmoid disease in FAP includes both desmoid reaction and desmoid tumors. Desmoid reaction is found within the abdomen in 13% of patients who have had a prior laparotomy [10]. It is a characteristic flat, white, hard sheet that is seen on the surface of the mesentery, often puckering the adjacent bowel (Fig. 8.1). While Clark et al. feel that the desmoid lesion is likely to be a precursor to a desmoid tumor [11], Hartley et al. found this not to be the case in 12 patients followed clinically for at least 4 years [10].

Desmoid tumors are mass lesions (Fig. 8.2) that can be defined in several ways.

1. Size: The largest diameter of desmoid tumors is measured on examination, at surgery, or on CT or MRI scanning. Comparative size is used to judge the response to treatment, and size is used in staging desmoids.
2. Location: 50% of FAP-related desmoid tumors occur within the abdomen, usually in the small bowel mesentery. About 45% are in the abdominal wall, some of which are associated with intra-abdominal extensions (i.e. transabdominal desmoids). A small proportion can be found in extra-abdominal locations, usually in patients with a 3′ *APC* mutation.

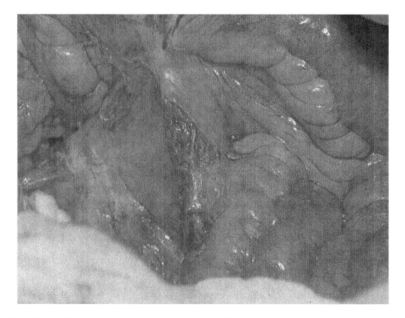

Fig. 8.1 Desmoid reaction: white sheets on the small bowel mesentery causing puckering and fixation of the bowel

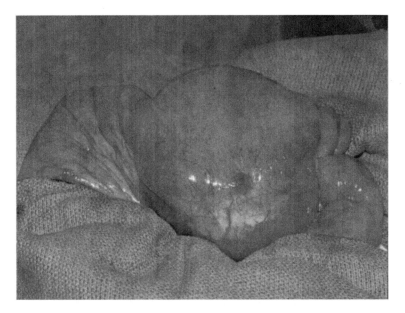

Fig. 8.2 Desmoid tumor in the small bowel mesentery

3. Behavior: Desmoids may be stable, shrink, or grow. Rapid growth can be defined as a change in maximum diameter of >50% in 3 months; slow growth is <50% change [12, 13].
4. Symptoms: Half of all desmoid disease is asymptomatic and is found incidentally either on CT scan or at laparotomy done for other reasons [14, 15]. Symptomatic desmoids present either as a mass, or with problems caused by their effect on adjacent organs: usually bowel or ureteric obstruction.

(Un)natural History

Most intra-abdominal desmoid tumors in FAP patients present within 4 years of their prophylactic surgery, be it colectomy and ileorectal anastomosis (IRA) or proctocolectomy and ileal pouch-anal anastomosis [6–8]. The usual presentation is with an abdominal mass or with symptoms of bowel or ureteric obstruction. CT scan of a desmoid tumor typically shows a homogenous mass lesion, although the only sign of the desmoid reaction may be stranding in the small bowel mesentery (Fig. 8.3). Tumor size can vary and, except for the extremes of size, bears little relationship to its ability to cause symptoms. Most desmoid tumors are either stable or grow very slowly [14]. Some shrink and disappear spontaneously while others grow rapidly and cause serious, sometimes lethal, problems (Fig. 8.4). Treatment is given for symptomatic or enlarging lesions.

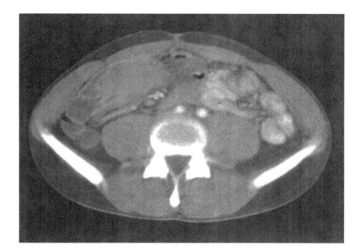

Fig. 8.3 Intra-abdominal desmoid tumor seen on CT scan

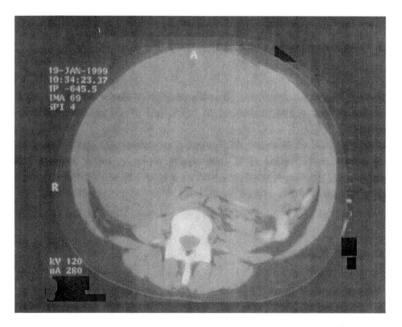

Fig. 8.4 Huge intra-abdominal desmoid seen on CT scan

Complications

The most common complications of desmoid disease are obstruction of either the small intestine or ureter. Small intestinal obstruction may require TPN but will sometimes resolve as the bowel adapts itself to the pressure effect of the slow-growing tumor. Ureteric obstruction is often treated with ureteric stents (Fig. 8.5). Stents are a temporary treatment and cause discomfort while predisposing to infection.

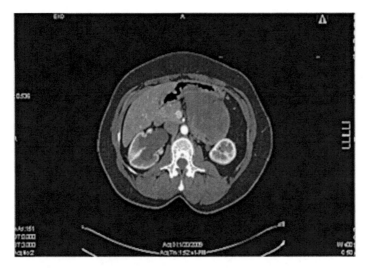

Fig. 8.5 Patient with ureteric obstruction due to a retroperitoneal desmoid, treated with ureteric stent

A more permanent urinary diversion is achieved with nephrostomy. Attempts at ureterolysis are ill-advised and can lead to an unplanned nephrectomy. The hope is that urinary diversion or stenting will be temporary while medical treatment causes the necessary softening or shrinkage of the desmoid. Recently, renal autotransplantation has emerged as an alternative to semi-permanent stenting, in patients whose abdomens are relatively friendly to surgeons. Table 8.1 shows the treatment of a series of 30 patients from the Cleveland Clinic with desmoid-related urinary tract involvement [16].

Desmoid tumors can erode into adjacent structures. The most frequent example is erosion into the bowel with development of an abscess and, ultimately, a fistula. The typical presentation is with fever and pain, CT scan showing a fluid and gas-filled cavity in the desmoid (Fig. 8.6). The differential diagnosis includes necrosis of the tumor with infection, or communication with an entrapped bowel loop. CT-guided drainage can relieve symptoms but may result in the development of a fistula. It is worth trying antibiotics prior to drainage, to see if a fistula can be avoided. Erosion into an adjacent artery can also occur and can be a terminal event.

Desmoid tumors may grow through a wound and present as an external mass (Fig. 8.7). These particularly aggressive tumors need urgent treatment, with antisarcoma chemotherapy, surgery, or radiation.

Predisposing Factors

Not every FAP patient will develop desmoid disease. Overall, symptomatic desmoid disease occurs in 12–15% of patients and asymptomatic desmoids are found in an additional 12–15% [10]. The tendency to develop desmoids is strongly

Table 8.1 Management of ureteric obstruction due to retroperitoneal desmoid disease in 30 patients with FAP (10 patients had >1 treatment)

Medications alone	9
Retrograde stenting	18
Nephrostomy +/– antegrade stent	5
Nephrectomy	4
Renal autotransplantation	3 (3 patients, 4 kidneys)
Ureterolysis	1
Ureteric resection and re-implantation	1

Source: Reprinted with permission from Ref. [16].

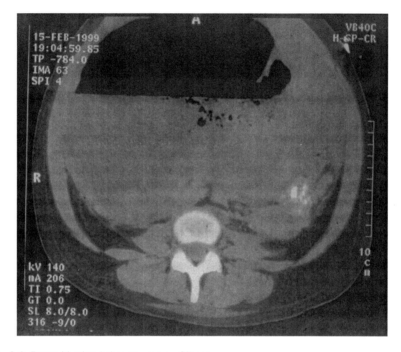

Fig. 8.6 Desmoid-related abscess seen on CT scan

related to genotype (discussed below) and gender. Although there are differences between series, women seem to be prone to develop desmoids. The worst behaving desmoids are those developing in young (early twenties), nulliparous women.

Surgery is the most common precipitating event leading to desmoid formation in desmoid-prone patients. Up to 80% of intra-abdominal desmoid disease is diagnosed postoperatively [10].

Recently a desmoid risk factor (DRF) was published that uses a formula based on gender, family history of desmoids, extracolonic manifestations of Gardner's syndrome and genotype to estimate an individual's risk for developing desmoid disease [17]. The Desmoid risk factor is shown in Table 8.2.

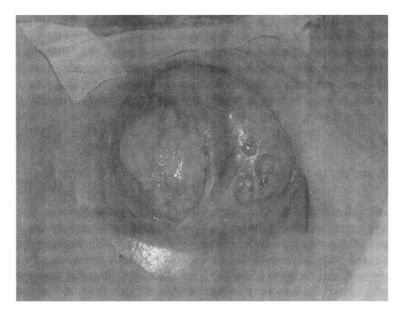

Fig. 8.7 Desmoid tumor growing through the abdominal wall

Table 8.2 Desmoid risk factor

Factors		Points		
		1	2	3
Gender		Male		Female
Family history		-ve	1	>1 relative
Extracolonic manifestations		0	1	>1
Genotype		<1,309	<1,900	>1,900
	With genotype	Without genotype		
Low risk	<7	<6		
Medium risk	7 to 8	6 to 7		
High risk	>8	>7		

Source: Reprinted with permission from Ref. [17]

Genetics

There is a strong correlation between *APC* genotype and desmoid predisposition. Several studies show that patients with their germline mutation located close to the 3′ end of exon 15 have an increased tendency to develop desmoid tumors [18–20]. There are at least three families in which desmoid disease is the predominant expression of the *APC* mutation and colorectal adenomatous polyposis is minimal or absent [21–24]. These families have mutations 3′ of codon 1900. Thus there is an inverse relationship between desmoid tendency and severity of polyposis.

In families with *APC* mutations in the more common loci at the 5' end of exon 15, desmoids are less common and the desmoid tendency less predictable.

The significance of the genotype–phenotype relationship of *APC* mutations and desmoids is that in some families a strong desmoid predisposition is either obvious or can be predicted. In these families there is a strong argument to delay the precipitating event, surgery, as long as is safe. Because the polyposis is usually mild, a delay of several years is often possible.

Relationship to Surgery

Desmoid disease is related to surgery in that surgery precipitates desmoids. However any relationship between the type or technique of surgery and risk of desmoid disease tends to be obscured by the relationship between desmoid tendency and polyposis severity. Thus, the stronger the desmoid tendency, the milder the polyposis, and the more likely that a colectomy and ileorectal anastomosis is performed. Severe polyposis is associated with a lesser desmoid risk and so a restorative proctocolectomy might be expected to be associated with lower risk of desmoids. This relationship argues against a common desire on the part of surgeons to "remove the rectum anyway so that later proctectomy, possibly made difficult or impossible by desmoids, will not be necessary." In fact, recent data from the Cleveland Clinic suggest that a laparoscopic restorative proctocolectomy is the surgical option most likely to produce clinically obvious desmoid disease. In descending order of "desmoidogenicity" were open restorative proctocolectomy, open colectomy and IRA and laparoscopic IRA [25]. The most likely explanation for this relationship of desmoids and surgical option is the increased tension on the small bowel mesentery resulting from an ileal pouch-anal anastomosis.

Desmoid disease may interfere with surgical strategy however. In most series of patients undergoing proctectomy or proctocolectomy for FAP there are a few patients in whom IPAA is impossible because of desmoids [10, 26, 27]. Desmoid disease shortens and tethers the ileal mesentery, preventing the pouch from reaching to the pelvic floor. Even if the pouch can be made, desmoids may prevent construction of a diverting ileostomy. Patients scheduled for proctectomy after prior colectomy need to be warned about this possibility.

Desmoids and Estrogens

The relationship between desmoid tumors and estrogen is both undeniable and ill-defined. It is suggested by the predominance of symptomatic desmoids in women and the tendency of aggressive, lethal desmoids to occur in young nulliparous women. Over 70% of desmoids express estrogen receptors [28], and there have been reports of enhanced desmoid growth during pregnancy [29, 30]. However there is also the observation that women who have been pregnant and develop desmoids have a significantly more benign course [31]. The paradox is that estrogens seem to both stimulate and inhibit desmoid disease. This is seen in the response of tumors to anti-estrogens, where some tumors regress and others grow. Overall, it seems as if a steady environment of relatively high levels of estrogens favors desmoids, but marked fluctuations in estrogen levels, either high or low, do not.

Diagnosis

Desmoid disease can be diagnosed in several different ways: on physical examination, where a hard mass is palpable within the abdominal wall or the abdomen itself; at surgery where the characteristic "white sheet" of the desmoid reaction is seen (Fig. 8.1), or where desmoid tumors present as hard white masses within the small bowel mesentery; and on CT scan, where mass lesions (Fig. 8.3) or even just a whorled appearance to the small bowel mesentery suggest desmoids [32]. In the right clinical setting (a patient with FAP), suggestive lesions do not need to be biopsied. Biopsies can be useful however, in confirming the diagnosis and in allowing tests for estrogen receptors or other proteins that may predict tumor behavior and response to treatment. Desmoid tumors should be measured objectively where possible. There has been a suggestion that enhancement of desmoids on the T2-weighted images of a magnetic resonance imaging scan predicts aggressive or active growth [33].

Staging

Desmoids differ in their presentation and behavior, and these differences may affect management decisions and the likely outcome of treatment. In order to stratify treatment by desmoid presentation, and to allow a meaningful analysis of outcome of treatment, a desmoid staging system has been proposed [15, 34]. This is system is shown in Table 8.3. Patients can move from stage to stage, either spontaneously or as a result of surgery or prior treatment [35]. The staging system has proved useful in separating patients by disease behavior and in analyzing the outcomes of surgery for abdominal desmoid disease in FAP [34, 35].

Management

There is no predictably effective treatment for desmoid disease. It is even difficult to find scientifically meaningful data about any potential agent because most reports are anecdotal or small retrospective series, and any prospective study is

Table 8.3 A staging system for intra-abdominal desmoid tumors [34]

Stage I	Asymptomatic disease, and not growing, and <10 cm in maximum diameter
Stage II	Minimally symptomatic, and not growing, or >10 cm in maximum diameter
Stage III	Symptomatic disease, or slowly growing, or obstructive complications
Stage IV	Symptomatic disease, and rapidly growing, or severe complications (e.g. fistula)

small and with inconclusive results [36]. There is no drug or combination of drugs that is clearly effective and that is an obvious first choice. There is weak evidence, however, showing some beneficial effect of nonsteroidal anti-inflammatory drugs (NSAIDs) [37–39], estrogen-blocking agents [40–45], combinations of nonsteroidal anti-inflammatory agents and estrogen-blocking drugs [46–50], and various chemotherapeutic drugs [51–57]. The recurrence rate after surgery is very high [58, 59], and although radiation is effective in treating a desmoid tumor [60, 61], its effects on adjacent bowel minimize its usefulness. The aim of treatment is not necessarily to make desmoid disease disappear but to render it stable and asymptomatic. Many patients with desmoids live with them for extended periods of time. Furthermore, some treatments used for desmoid disease have significant toxicity, so that the treatment needs to be appropriate for the severity of the presentation.

Stage I Disease

Treatment for asymptomatic disease is largely prophylactic and there are no data to determine its real need. While the St Marks group suggests that the flat desmoid "precursor" lesion is at risk for becoming clinically problematic [11, 62], the Cleveland Clinic data show that this is not the case [10]. However asymptomatic desmoid tumors can grow and cause problems, so there is a case for treating them. Currently the nonsteroidal anti-inflammatory drug (NSAID) clinoril (Sulindac) is commonly used [38, 39]. There is evidence from a retrospective controlled study that clinoril has some activity against desmoids [12], although the response may be very slow. Side effects of clinoril (dose 150–200 mg twice daily with food) include gastric distress, gastrointestinal ulcerations, renal toxicity and bleeding from platelet dysfunction.

Stage II Disease

Mildly symptomatic or relatively large, asymptomatic desmoid tumors are usually treated with a NSAID, an estrogen-blocking agent, or a combination of the two. The response to high dose tamoxifen in combination with sulindac in one recent German study has been good, with 18/18 patients having some reduction in tumor size or symptoms after treatment with a maximum dose of 120 mg/day [46]. Raloxifene, an estrogen-blocking agent with fewer side effects than tamoxifen, was also effective in inducing either a total or partial response in all patients in the one study reported so far [45]. There were initially hopes of success with the use of toremifene, also an estrogen-blocking drug [42–44]. However, the Cleveland Clinic stopped enrolling into a toremifene trial because of evidence that tumors grew faster when the patient was on toremifene (unpublished data).

Stage III Disease

Estrogen blockade is often the first choice treatment for patients with enlarging desmoids in whom an urgent response is not needed. High dose tamoxifen (increased in steps up to 120 mg/day) or raloxifene (120 mg/day) may be used. Alternatives include the chemotherapy combination of vinorelbine/vinblastine and methotrexate, although this is not as predictably effective [55–57]. Other drugs which have been reported as case reports or tiny series are the anti-fibrosis agent pirfenidone [63], interferon alpha [64, 65] and Gleevac [66, 67]. Recent data from the Cleveland Clinic reporting strong expression of VEGF and EGF receptors in desmoid tumors suggest a role for the antibodies bevacizumab and erbitux [68], but no reliable data are yet available regarding their efficacy.

Stage IV Disease

Desmoid tumors that are growing rapidly are a threat to life, and need urgently to be brought under control. The best way of treating such tumors is with anti-sarcoma therapy, adriamycin, dacarbazine, and cisplatinum. Such extremely toxic therapy carries its own mortality, but has been shown to produce rapid regression in some tumors and at least a partial response in the majority [51–54]. Recently the liposonal form of doxorubicin (Doxil) has been reported to be effective [72].

Surgery

Most intra-abdominal desmoid tumors involve the root of the small bowel mesentery, and attempts at resection often result in loss of large amounts of small intestine [58, 59]. There is at least one report of total enterectomy and small bowel transplant in 12 patients with FAP-associated desmoids [70]. Unfortunately the recurrence rate of abdominal desmoids is over 50%, making the value of such surgical extravaganzas questionable. Occasionally, however, a mesenteric desmoid is peripheral enough to allow resection with removal of only a small amount of bowel (Fig. 8.2). Sometimes desmoids can be resected while preserving an ileal pouch [71], although this is likely to be rare. Patients undergoing surgery for excision of desmoids need to be aware that they may end up with a permanent ileostomy.

Surgery for intra-abdominal desmoids is therefore rarely elective. It is a last resort, where all else has failed or when there is a life-threatening complication. Abdominal wall desmoids are a different matter however. Here resection with free margins is much more likely, and the prospect of extensive bowel resection is small. Excision of large tumors leaves large defects in the abdominal wall that must be close with abdominal wall reconstruction. Therefore, aggressive surgery for abdominal wall desmoids, removing them before they grow too large, is indicated. Transabdominal desmoids are particularly dangerous, as their abdominal wall component may be resected and commit the surgeon to resect a complex and difficult retroperitoneal and mesenteric component.

Radiation

Desmoid tumors are radio-sensitive [60, 61], but when in the abdomen, they are usually too close to bowel loops for the radiation to be given safely. Radiation can be used where its dosage can be confined to the tumor. This suggests the intra-operative radiation may be worth trying in the context of unresectable tumors.

Treating the Family

Desmoid disease can be catastrophic in patients and families with FAP. Because the incidence and severity of the disease is related to genotype some families are particularly prone to the almost inevitable disasters that lie in wait for them. It is difficult to watch a close relative die unpleasantly because of desmoid disease, and to know that you have the same predisposition. Hence the attitude of delaying colectomy indefinitely in families where desmoid disease is particularly severe is justifiable, as long as the risk of colorectal cancer is low. Chemoprevention with sulindac may not only minimize colonic disease but also suppress desmoid tendency.

Summary

Desmoid disease occurs in 31% of patients with FAP, mostly appearing after the index abdominal surgery. Patients are predisposed to desmoid formation by their genotype and gender, and this predisposition usually shows up in the family. Untreated, a minority of desmoids grow and some are lethal, especially when they occur in young, nulliparous women. Most desmoids never threaten life and cause intermittent symptoms of abdominal pain or bowel obstruction. Although there are multiple treatment options, no single treatment is satisfactory in every patient. The best treatment strategy for intra-abdominal tumors is to begin with the least toxic medical treatment and to work through increasingly toxic options if there is no response. Surgery is usually a last resort for intra-abdominal desmoids.

References

1. Reitamo JJ, Hayry P, Nykyri E, Saxen E. The desmoid tumor. I. Incidence, sex-, age- and anatomical distribution in the Finnish population. Am J Clin Pathol 1982;77:665–73.
2. Lips DJ, Barker N, Clevers H, Hennipman A. The role of APC and beta-catenin in the aetiology of aggressive fibromatosis (desmoid tumors). Eur J Surg Oncol 2009 Jan;35(1):3–10.
3. Tejpar S, Michils G, Denys H, Van Dam K, Nik SA, Jadidizadeh A, Cassiman JJ. Analysis of Wnt/Beta catenin signalling in desmoid tumors. Acta Gastroenterol Belg 2005 Jan-Mar;68(1):5–9.
4. Ballo MT, Zagars GK, Pollack A, Pisters PW, Pollack RA. Desmoid tumor: prognostic factors and outcome after surgery, radiation therapy, or combined surgery and radiation therapy. J Clin Oncol 1999;17(1):158–67.
5. Duggal A, Dickinson IC, Sommerville S, Gallie P. The management of extra-abdominal desmoid tumours. Int Orthop 2004;28:252–6.
6. Clark SK, Neale KF, Landgrebe JC, Phillips RK. Desmoid tumours complicating familial adenomatous polyposis. Br J Surg 1999;86:1185–9.
7. Soravia C, Berk T, McLeod RS, Cohen Z. Desmoid disease in patients with familial adenomatous polyposis. Dis Colon Rectum 2000;43:363–9.
8. Rodriguez-Bigas MA, Mahoney MC, Karakousis CP, Petrelli NJ. Desmoid tumors in patients with familial adenomatous polyposis. Cancer 1994;74:1270–4.
9. Arvanitis ML, Jagelman DG, Fazio VW, Lavery IC, McGannon E. Mortality in patients with familial adenomatous polyposis. Dis Colon Rectum 1990;33:639–42.
10. Hartley JE, Church JM, Gupta S, McGannon E, Fazio VW. Significance of incidental desmoids identified during surgery for familial adenomatous polyposis. Dis Colon Rectum 2004;47:334–8.
11. Clark SK, Smith TG, Katz DE, Reznek RH, Phillips RK. Identification and progression of a desmoid precursor lesion in patients with familial adenomatous polyposis. Br J Surg 1998;85:970–3.
12. Tsukada K, Church JM, Jagelman DG, Fazio VW, McGannon E, George CR, Schroeder T, Lavery I, Oakley J. Noncytotoxic drug therapy for intra-abdominal desmoid tumor in patients with familial adenomatous polyposis. Dis Colon Rectum 1992;35:29–33.
13. Tsukada K, Church JM, Jagelman DG, Fazio VW, Lavery IC. Systemic cytotoxic chemotherapy and radiation therapy for desmoid in familial adenomatous polyposis. Dis Colon Rectum 1991;34:1090–2.
14. Lynch AC, Ozuner G, Church JM. The clinical course of desmoid tumors in familial adenomatous polyposis. Dis Colon Rectum 2003;46:A53.
15. Church J, Berk T, Boman B, et al. Staging intra-abdominal desmoid tumors in familial adenomatous polyposis; a search for a uniform approach to a troubling disease. Dis Colon Rectum 2005;48:1528–34.
16. Mignanelli E, Joyce M, Church J. Ureteric obstruction. Dis Colon Rectum 2009;52: 811.
17. Elayi E, Manilich E, Church J. Polishing the crystal ball: knowing genotype improves ability to predict desmoid disease. Dis Colon Rectum 2008;51:802–3.
18. Bertario L, Russo A, Sala P, et al. Hereditary Colorectal Tumours Registry. Genotype and phenotype factors as determinants of desmoid tumors in patients with familial adenomatous polyposis. Int J Cancer 2001;95:102–7.
19. Friedl W, Caspari R, Sengteller M et al. Can APC mutation analysis contribute to therapeutic decisions in familial adenomatous polyposis? Experience from 680 FAP families. Gut 2001;48:515–21.
20. Bunyan DJ, Shea-Simonds J, Reck AC, Finnis D, Eccles DM. Genotype-phenotype correlations of new causative APC gene mutations in patients with familial adenomatous polyposis. J Med Genet 1995;32:728–31.
21. Scott RJ, Froggatt NJ, Trembath RC et al. Familial infiltrative fibromatosis (desmoid tumours) (MIM135290) caused by a recurrent 3' APC gene mutation. Hum Mol Genet 1996;5:1921–4.

22. Eccles DM, van der Luijt R, Breukel C et al. Hereditary desmoid disease due to a frameshift mutation at codon 1924 of the APC gene. Am J Hum Genet 1996;59:1193–201.
23. Matsubara N, Isozaki H, Tanaka N. The farthest 3' distal end APC mutation identified in attenuated adenomatous polyposis coli with extracolonic manifestations. Dis Colon Rectum 2000;43:720–1.
24. Couture J, Mitri A, Lagace R et al. A germline mutation at the extreme 3' end of the APC gene results in a severe desmoid phenotype and is associated with overexpression of beta-catenin in the desmoid tumor. Clin Genet 2000;57:205–12.
25. Vogel J, Church JM, LaGuardia L. Minimally invasive pouch surgery predisposes to desmoid tumor formation in patients with familial adenomatous polyposis. Dis Colon Rectum 2005;48:662
26. Penna C, Tiret E, Parc R et al. Operation and abdominal desmoid tumors in familial adenomatous polyposis. Surg Gynecol Obstet 1993;177:263–268
27. Browning SM, Nivatvongs S. Intraoperative abandonment of ileal pouch to anal anastomosis-the Mayo Clinic experience. J Am Coll Surg 1998;186:441–5.
28. Lim CL, Walker MJ, Mehta RR, Das Gupta TK. Estrogen and anti-estrogen binding sites in desmoid tumors. Eur J Cancer Clin Oncol 1986; 22: 583–7.
29. Mulik V, Griffiths AN, Beattie RB. Desmoid tumours with familial adenomatous polyposis in pregnancy. J Obstet Gynaecol 2003;23:307–8.
30. Way JC, Culham BA. Desmoid tumour. The risk of recurrent or new disease with subsequent pregnancy: a case report. Can J Surg 1999;42:51–4.
31. Church JM, McGannon E. Prior pregnancy ameliorates the course of intra-abdominal desmoid tumors in patients with familial adenomatous polyposis. Dis Colon Rectum 2000;43:445–50.
32. Brooks AP, Reznek RH, Nugent K, Farmer KC, Thomson JP, Phillips RK. CT appearances of desmoid tumours in familial adenomatous polyposis: further observations. Clin Radiol 1994;49(9):601–7
33. Healy JC, Reznek RH, Clark SK, Phillips RK, Armstrong P. MR appearances of desmoid tumors in familial adenomatous polyposis. AJR Am J Roentgenol. 1997;169(2):465–72.
34. Church J, Lynch C, Neary P, LaGuardia L, Elayi E. A desmoid tumor-staging system separates patients with intra-abdominal, familial adenomatous polyposis-associated desmoid disease by behavior and prognosis. Dis Colon Rectum 2008;51:897–901.
35. Church J, Elayi E, and Xhaja X. Outcomes of surgery for abdominal desmoid tumors in FAP Hered Ca Clin Pract 2010 in press.
36. Lindor NM, Dozois R, Nelson H et al. Desmoid tumors in familial adenomatous polyposis: a pilot project evaluating the efficacy of treatment with pirfenidone. Am L Gastroenterol 2003;98:1868–74.
37. Lackner H, Urban C, Kerbl R, Schwinger W, Beham A. Noncytotoxic drug therapy in children with unresectable desmoid tumors. Cancer 1997;80(2):334–40.
38. D'Alteroche L, Benchellal ZA, Salem N, Regimbeau C, Picon L, Metman EH. Complete remission of a mesenteric fibromatosis after taking sulindac Gastroenterol Clin Biol 1998;22:1098–101.
39. Belliveau P, Graham AM. Mesenteric desmoid tumor in Gardner's syndrome treated by sulindac. Dis Colon Rectum 1984;27:53–4.
40. Maroy B. Desmoid tumor sensitive to tamoxifen Presse Med 1997;26:1520–2
41. Chao AS, Lai CH, Hsueh S, Chen CS, Yang YC, Soong YK. Successful treatment of recurrent pelvic desmoid tumour with tamoxifen: case report Hum Reprod 2000;15:311–3.
42. Brooks MD, Ebbs SR, Colletta AA, Baum M. Desmoid tumours treated with triphenylethylenes Eur J Cancer 1992;28A(6–7):1014–8.
43. Benson JR, Mokbel K, Baum M. Management of desmoid tumours including a case report of toremifene. Ann Oncol 1994;5(2):173–7.
44. Bus PJ, Verspaget HW, van Krieken JH, de Roos A, Keizer HJ, Bemelman WA, Vasen HF, Lamers CB, Griffioen G. Treatment of mesenteric desmoid tumours with the anti-oestrogenic agent toremifene: case histories and an overview of the literature. Eur J Gastroenterol Hepatol 1999;11:1179–83.

45. Tonelli F, Ficari F, Valanzano R, Brandi ML. Treatment of desmoids and mesenteric fibromatosis in familial adenomatous polyposis with raloxifene. Tumori 2003;89:391–6.
46. Hansmann A, Adolph C, Vogel T, Unger A, Moslein G. High-dose tamoxifen and sulindac as first-line treatment for desmoid tumors. Cancer 2004;100:612–20.
47. Clark SK. Sulindac and tamoxifen in the treatment of desmoid tumours in patients with familial adenomatous polyposis. Colorectal Dis 2002;4:68.
48. Bulow S. Sulindac and tamoxifen in the treatment of desmoid tumours in patients with familial adenomatous polyposis. Colorectal Dis 2001;3:266–7.
49. Izes JK, Zinman LN, Larsen CR. Regression of large pelvic desmoid tumor by tamoxifen and sulindac. Urology 1996;47:756–9.
50. Klein WA, Miller HH, Anderson M, DeCosse JJ. The use of indomethacin, sulindac, and tamoxifen for the treatment of desmoid tumors associated with familial polyposis. Cancer 1987;60(12):2863–8.
51. Seiter K, Kemeny N. Successful treatment of a desmoid tumor with doxorubicin Cancer 1993 71:2242–4.
52. Lynch HT, Fitzgibbons R Jr, Chong S, Cavalieri J, Lynch J, Wallace F, Patel S. Use of doxorubicin and dacarbazine for the management of unresectable intra-abdominal desmoid tumors in Gardner's syndrome. Dis Colon Rectum 1994;37:260–7.
53. Schnitzler M, Cohen Z, Blackstein M, Berk T, Gallinger S, Madlensky L, McLeod R. Chemotherapy for desmoid tumors in association with familial adenomatous polyposis. Dis Colon Rectum 1997;40:798–801.
54. Poritz LS, Blackstein M, Berk T, Gallinger S, McLeod RS, Cohen Z. Extended follow-up of patients treated with cytotoxic chemotherapy for intra-abdominal desmoid tumors Dis Colon Rectum 2001;44:1268–73.
55. Azzarelli A, Gronchi A, Bertulli R, Tesoro JD, Baratti D, Pennacchioli E, Dileo P, Rasponi A, Ferrari A, Pilotti S, Casali PG. Low-dose chemotherapy with methotrexate and vinblastine for patients with advanced aggressive fibromatosis. Cancer. 2001;92(5):1259–64.
56. Weiss AJ, Horowitz S, Lackman RD. Therapy of desmoid tumors and fibromatosis using vinorelbine. Am J Clin Oncol 1999;22(2):193–5.
57. Kono T, Tomita I, Chisato N, Matsuda M, Kakisaka A, Kasai S. Successful low-dose chemotherapy using vinblastine and methotrexate for the treatment of an ileoanal pouch mesenteric desmoid tumor: report of a case. Dis Colon Rectum 2004;47(2):246–9.
58. Middleton SB, Phillips RK. Surgery for large intra-abdominal desmoid tumors: report of four cases. Dis Colon Rectum 2000;43:1759–62
59. Smith AJ, Lewis JJ, Merchant NB, Leung DH, Woodruff JM, Brennan MF. Surgical management of intra-abdominal desmoid tumours. Br J Surg 2000;87:608–13.
60. Jelinek JA, Stelzer KJ, Conrad E, et al. The efficacy of radiotherapy as postoperative treatment for desmoid tumors. Int J Rad Oncol Biol Phys 2001;50:121–5.
61. Nuyttens JJ, Rust PF, Thomas CR Jr, Turrisi AT 3rd. Surgery versus radiation therapy for patients with aggressive fibromatosis or desmoid tumors: A comparative review of 22 articles. Cancer 2000; 88:1517–23.
62. Middleton SB, Clark SK, Matravers P, Katz D, Reznek R, Phillips RK. Stepwise progression of familial adenomatous polyposis-associated desmoid precursor lesions demonstrated by a novel CT scoring system. Dis Colon Rectum 2003;46:481–5.
63. Lindor NM, Dozois R, Nelson H, Wolff B, King J, Boardman L, Wilson M, Greene MH, Karnes W, Mesa R, Welch T, Edmonson J, Limburg P. Desmoid tumors in familial adenomatous polyposis: a pilot project evaluating efficacy of treatment with pirfenidone. Am J Gastroenterol 2003;98(8):1868–74
64. Hardell L, Breivald M, Hennerdal S, Fernberg JO, Strander H. Shrinkage of desmoid tumor with interferon alfa treatment: a case report. Cytokines Cell Mol Ther 2000;6(3):155–6.
65. Tjandra SS, Hsu C, Goh YI, Gurung A, Poon R, Nadesan P, Alman BA. IFN-{beta} signaling positively regulates tumorigenesis in aggressive fibromatosis, potentially by modulating mesenchymal progenitors. Cancer Res 2007;67(15):7124–31.

66. Ravaioli A, Nicoletti S, Tamburini E, Papi M. Control of aggressive fibromatosis by treatment with imatinib mesylate: a step forward? J Cancer Res Clin Oncol 2009;135(2):325–6.
67. Wcislo G, Szarlej-Wcislo K, Szczylik C.Control of aggressive fibromatosis by treatment with imatinib mesylate. A case report and review of the literature. J Cancer Res Clin Oncol 2007;133(8):533–8.
68. Vogel J, Schade A, Goldblum J, Yerian L, Church J. New hope for patients with FAP-associated desmoids: vascular endothelial growth factor receptor and epithelial growth factor receptorare expressed in most tumors. Dis Colon Rectum 2006;49:753.
69. Latchford AR, Sturt NJ, Neale K, Rogers PA, Phillips RK. A 10-year review of surgery for desmoid disease associated with familial adenomatous polyposis. Br J Surg 2006;93(10):1258–64
70. Chatzipetrou MA, Tzakis AG, Pinna AD, Kato T, Misiakos EP, Tsaroucha AK, Weppler D, Ruiz P, Berho M, Fishbein T, Conn HO, Ricordi C. Intestinal transplantation for the treatment of desmoid tumors associated with familial adenomatous polyposis. Surgery 2001;129(3):277–81.
71. Guy RJ, Mortensen NJ. Successful resection of an ileoanal pouch mesenteric desmoid without pouch sacrifice: report of a case. Dis Colon Rectum 2000;43(5):713–6.
72. Bertagnolli MM, Morgan JA, Fletcher CD, Raut CP, Dileop, Gill RR et al. Multimodality treatment of mesenteric desmoid tumors Eur J Ca 2008; 44:2404–10.

Chapter 9
Hereditary Nonpolyposis Colorectal Cancer

W. Donald Buie and Anthony R. MacLean

Hereditary nonpolyposis colorectal cancer (HNPCC) is one of two distinct inherited colorectal cancer syndromes with known genetic defects. It is estimated to account for approximately 5% of all large bowel cancers. Originally called Lynch syndrome after Dr. Henry Lynch, it is an autosomal dominant disorder characterized by a predilection for colorectal cancer and other secondary cancers in affected individuals. Although initially separated into Lynch I (families with colorectal cancer alone) and Lynch II (families with colorectal cancer associated with other secondary cancers), this distinction does not conform to genotypic differences but appears to be due to phenotypic variation. Subsequently, the name HNPCC was formulated to differentiate it from familial adenomatous polyposis (FAP) syndrome. Unfortunately this name is misleading as these patients do form polyps (although to a lesser degree than in FAP) and it does not acknowledge the secondary cancers which are an important part of this syndrome. Recently, there has been a trend back toward the use of Lynch syndrome to describe this entity.

History

The first study of a family that had what is now known as Lynch syndrome or HNPCC began in 1895 [1]. Dr. Aldred Warthin, a well-known pathologist, learned that his seamstress was convinced she would die at an early age because of a cancer of the female organs or bowels, because everyone in her family died of those cancers. She did go on to die of metastatic endometrial cancer at an early age, and Warthin subsequently published a description of her family, which he called Family G, in 1913 [1].

About 50 years passed before a resident in internal medicine, Dr. Henry Lynch, met a patient with delirium tremens. The man was questioned about his drinking,

W.D. Buie (✉)
Department of Surgery, Division of General Surgery, University of Calgary, Calgary, Canada
and
1403 29th St., NW Calgary, Alberta Canada T3H 1L8
e-mail: wdbuie@ucalgary.ca

C.N. Ellis (ed.), *Inherited Cancer Syndromes: Current Clinical Management*,
DOI 10.1007/978-1-4419-6821-0_9, © Springer Science+Business Media, LLC 2011

and revealed that he, like everyone in his family, was going to die of cancer, most likely colon cancer. Dr. Lynch went on to compile this man's family history. Many family members reported a history of cancer, particularly colon cancer, and often at an early age. Among the women there was also a high rate of endometrial and ovarian cancers. A review of the literature did not find any evidence of a hereditary basis for this combination of cancers, and Lynch wondered whether they were dealing with a new hereditary cancer syndrome. The family was labeled Family N, for Nebraska. He went on to collect medical and pathologic information on the affected family members, and noted that in the cases of colon cancers, there was no evidence of multiple colonic polyps to suggest FAP.

Dr. Lynch presented the kindred in 1964 at the American Society of Human Genetics, and during that presentation Dr. Marjorie Shaw mentioned that she had studied a similar kindred in Michigan, which she called Family M. She invited Lynch and his colleagues to study this family. They went on to publish their findings on these two kindreds in 1966 [2].

Lynch and colleagues then began studying other cancer prone families and reviewing the literature of families whose cancer findings were suggestive of a hereditary cancer syndrome. Based on these families, in 1971 Lynch reported the criteria for the "cancer family syndrome," which consisted of an increased incidence of adenocarcinomas, particularly of the colon and endometrium, an increased frequency of multiple primary malignancies, an early age of onset, and an auto-somal dominant inheritance pattern [3]. Further study allowed Lynch to add that the colon cancers in Lynch syndrome had a predilection for the ascending colon, with about one-third of them occurring in the cecum [4].

In an effort to improve the identification of kindreds at risk for HNPCC, a group of world experts which came to be known as the International Collaborative Group (ICG) on HNPCC met in Amsterdam in August of 1990, and among other things established the minimum criteria for the identification of HNPCC, now known as the Amsterdam Criteria [5]. Because these criteria do not account for small kindreds or the extraco-lonic HNPCC-associated cancers, the National Cancer Institute convened an interna-tional expert panel in November 1996 in Bethesda, Maryland to clarify the role of genetics in the pathology of HNPCC [6]. Discussions included strategies to identify potential HNPCC patients not identified by the Amsterdam Criteria. Guidelines were established for testing colorectal cancers for microsatellite instability, which have been termed the Bethesda Criteria. The ICG had further discussions at their ninth and tenth annual meetings to further refine the original Amsterdam Criteria, to make the criteria more sensitive for the detection of HNPCC. These discussions culminated in the estab-lishment of the Amsterdam II Criteria, published in 1999 [7].

Much of our current understanding of the molecular genetics of HNPCC was described in 1993 and 1994. Aaltonen et al. first described the "replication error phenotype" [8], now known as microsatellite instability. Linkage analysis identified a site on genes 2P [9] and 3P [10] as loci for the genes responsible for HNPCC. Mutations in the hMLH-1 and hMSH-2 were subsequently identified [11–13]. Additional genes have since been identified, including hMSH-6 [14], hPMS-1, hPMS-2 [15], and hMSH-3 [16].

Definition

While there is no absolute definition that establishes the diagnosis of HNPCC, there are several features that are commonly seen. These include an autosomal pattern of inheritance with penetrance of approximately 90%, early age of onset, proximal location of colonic cancers, frequent synchronous and metachronous colorectal cancers, better prognosis than in sporadic cases stage for stage, and increased risk of certain extra-colonic malignancies. Pathologic features include poor differentiation, increased signet ring cells, medullary subtype, and tumor infiltrating lymphocytes or Crohn's-like reaction, as well as a high frequency of MSI-H, loss of expression of DNA mismatch repair proteins on immunohistochemistry, and a germline mutation in one of the DNA mismatch repair genes.

Clinical Manifestations

Age of Onset

Patients with HNPCC-associated colorectal cancer tend to present at an earlier age than those with sporadic colorectal cancer. Males and females with sporadic cancer present at a median age of 70.7 and 74.2 years, respectively [17], whereas in patients with HNPCC-associated colorectal cancer, the median age at presentation is approximately 45 years of age [18–20], or about 25 years younger than sporadic cases.

Tumor Distribution

While greater than 50% of sporadic cancers are located in the rectum or sigmoid colon, approximately 70% of HNPCC-associated cancers are seen proximal to the splenic flexure [18]. In a study by Lin et al. over 40% of HNPCC cancers were in the right colon, compared to only 25% of sporadic cancers [20].

Synchronous and Metachronous Tumors

The rate of synchronous cancers in patients with HNPCC-associated colorectal cancer is approximately 7%, compared to 2.5% in sporadic cases [20], while the annual risk of metachronous cancers is approximately 2% in HNPCC patients, compared to 0.3% in sporadic patients. In addition, of all patients with synchronous colorectal cancers, the rate of MSI is approximately 35% [21].

Table 9.1 Extra-colonic HNPCC-associated cancers and their screening recommendations

Site	Risk of malignancy (%)	Screening option	Age to begin screening	Interval
Endometrial	27–72	Gynecologic examination Transvaginal ultrasound Endometrial biopsy (can consider prophylactic hysterectomy)	30–35	1–2
Ovarian	3–13			

Gastric	2–13	Consider if family history of gastric
		    cancer or if from country with
		    high incidence of gastric cancer
		Upper GI endoscopy
			30–35	1–2

Small bowel	4–7			
Hepatobiliary	2			1–2
Renal pelvis/ ureteric	1–12	Abdominal ultrasound Urinalysis, urine cytology		1–2
Brain tumor	1–4			

Extra-colonic Tumors

There is an increased risk of several extra-colonic cancers in kindreds with HNPCC (see Table 9.1). Extra-colonic cancers include endometrial, ovarian, gastric, small bowel, hepatobiliary, brain, renal pelvis/ureteric, and skin neoplasms, including sebaceous adenoma, sebaceous adenocarcinoma, and multiple keratoacanthomas. The risk of these extracolonic malignancies varies depending upon the affected kindred, and no screening regime has proven thus far to be cost effective or to change the patient outcome. Despite this, several screening strategies exist, and their implementation, particularly in patients with a family history of any of these cancers, may be of some benefit (see Screening section).

Stage at Presentation

While different groups have reported differing proportions of patients in each stage at presentation, in general HNPCC tumors have lower rates of presenting with stage 4 disease [20, 22].

Molecular Genetics and Histopathology

DNA Mismatch Repair

As cells prepare to divide, they replicate their DNA. Errors, or mismatches, may occur during replication, usually on long, repeating nucleotide sequences called microsatellites. Errors in DNA replication are usually identified and repaired by proteins known as the mismatch repair proteins. The hMSH-2 protein combines with the hMSH-6 and hMSH-3 proteins to form an active mismatch repair protein that identifies areas in the DNA where replication errors have been made. The hMLH-1 protein, meanwhile, combines with the hPMS-2 protein to form an active complex that actually carries out the repair. The repairs occur by removing the segment of DNA containing the errors, and replacing it with a corrected DNA sequence.

At least 40% of the identified gene mutations in patients with HNPCC occur in hMSH-2. Several hundred different mutations of this gene have been described. These mutations can cause a short or inactive hMSH-2 protein, so that it cannot perform its usual function. This allows DNA replication errors to go unnoticed and therefore unrepaired. Mutations in hMSH-6 or hMSH-3 cause a similar malfunction in the active protein that detects replication errors. This results in the accumulation of DNA errors, eventually causing mutations of tumor suppressor genes, or other genes that control cell division, resulting in neoplastic transformation. Genes at particular risk are those that contain microsatellites, including TGFBIIR, BAX, Caspase, hMSH-3, and hMSH-6.

Another 40% or more of identified gene mutations occur in hMLH-1. As with hMSH-2, there have been several hundred described mutations in hMLH-1. These mutations also cause a short or inactive hMLH-1 protein that is unable to function normally. Thus, DNA replication errors cannot be repaired, leading to the accumulation of DNA errors, again leading to neoplastic development. Mutations in hPMS-2 cause a similar problem in DNA replication error repair.

Patients with a homozygous mutation of one of the mismatch repair proteins develop a distinct syndrome from HNPCC, with leukemias or lymphomas, neurofibromatosis, and early onset colorectal cancer [23].

Microsatellites and Microsatellite Instability

Microsatellites are polymorphic loci in nuclear DNA that consist of repeating units of 1–4 bases in length, which are often repeated 10–100 times. Microsatellites have a high rate of variability thanks to a high rate of mutations, compared to other areas of DNA. This high rate of mutations is thought to occur by slipped strand mispairing during DNA replication. When mutations in the DNA mismatch repair genes are present, these sequences become shorter or longer. The occurrence of long or short microsatellites in a person's DNA is referred to as microsatellite instability and is a marker for DNA mismatch repair.

When a DNA microsatellite error goes unrecognized or unrepaired, as occurs in HNPCC, frameshift mutations can occur in key tumor suppressor genes, causing them to malfunction or become inactivated, leading to neoplastic transformation. Another mechanism where MSI can cause colorectal cancer is by a frameshift mutation causing a mutation in an essential mismatch repair gene, resulting in the accumulation of further DNA replication errors.

Many variations on the definition of microsatellite instability have been proposed. A consensus conference established specific guidelines for testing. A reference panel of five microsatellites are tested in colorectal cancer (BAT 25, BAT 26, D2S123,

D5S346, and D18S69 or D17S250), and tumors are classified as having high-frequency microsatellite instability if two or more of the five markers show instability compared to normal tissue from the same patient, as low frequency microsatellite instability if one of the five markers shows instability, and as microsatellite stable if no markers have instability.

Approximately 15% of sporadic colorectal cancer and close to 90% of HNPCC-associated colorectal cancers have microsatellite instability. Of the 15% of sporadic colorectal cancers, some will prove to have a mutation of one of the mismatch repair genes, but the majority will have methylation of the hMLH-1 gene. Methylation occurs in the promoter region of the 5' end of a gene; promoter methylation silences the gene so that no protein is made, and in this case identified errors of DNA replication cannot be repaired.

Immunohistochemistry

Immunohistochemistry can be very useful in identifying the mutated gene in cases that are suspicious for a mismatch repair deficiency. The loss of expression of MSH-2 or MSH-6 proteins is virtually diagnostic of HNPCC, since virtually all of the sporadic cases of MSI-H tumors will have loss of expression of MLH-1 due to methylation. When loss of a mismatch repair protein is demonstrated, germline testing can be focused on that gene, and in the case of MLH-1, testing for methylation can be carried out.

Histopathology

The most important histologic feature for predicting HNPCC is lymphocytic infiltration. Patterns of lymphocytic infiltration include a nodular or Crohn's-like peritumoral lymphocytic reaction, and tumor-infiltrating lymphocytes. Other features that have been identified in MSI-H cancers include poor differentiation, mucinous differentiation, medullary type adenocarcinomas, lower frequency of lymph node metastases, and lower frequency of DNA aneuploidy.

Clinical Recognition

Differences from Familial Adenomatous Polyposis

While differentiating HNPCC from conventional FAP is usually fairly straightforward, patients with attenuated FAP may be more difficult to sort out. Typical FAP patients have greater than 100 adenomas, with early onset of adenomas, occasionally even in preteen years, with cancer occurring in most patients by 40 or 50 years of age. Likewise, extra-colonic features of FAP also differ from HNPCC. FAP extra-colonic features include gastric, duodenal and peri-ampullary adenomas, desmoids tumors, papillary thyroid cancers, hepatoblastomas, medulloblastomas, sarcomas, pancreatic carcinomas, osteomas, and congenital hypertrophy of the retinal pigment epithelium (CHRPE). From a molecular standpoint, FAP is characterized by a mutation of the APC gene, whereas HNPCC tumors are associated with MSI.

Attenuated FAP (aFAP) patients can be more difficult to distinguish from HNPCC. They have fewer adenomas (<100), adenomas are more commonly seen proximal to the splenic flexure, and neoplasms present at an age more in keeping with HNPCC. In addition, desmoids and CHRPE are absent in aFAP. However, gastric fundic polyps and duodenal adenomas are commonly seen.

HNPCC Criteria

A number of guidelines have been established to help with the clinical recognition of patients with HNPCC (see Table 9.2). Each has its own pitfalls, and as the sensitivity of the guidelines has improved, so too has the specificity declined. The Amsterdam criteria originally published in 1991 were found to be 60% sensitive and 70% specific in identifying patients with germline mutations of hMLH-1 or hMSH-2. The Amsterdam II criteria increased the sensitivity to 78%, but decreased the specificity to 61%. The Bethesda and modified Bethesda criteria meanwhile increased the sensitivity to about 90%, but also decreased the specificity to approximately 20% [24, 25].

Another option to identify patients with HNPCC is to evaluate all patients with colorectal cancer according to the guideline published by Hampel et al. [26] Basically, all tumors would get evaluated using immunohistochemistry for hMLH-1, hMSH-2, hMSH-6, and hPMS-2. Those that stain for all proteins would have no further testing. Those with no staining of hMLH-1 and hPMS-2 would be evaluated for Methylation of hMLH-1 promoter. If there is no evidence of Methylation, the gene would get sequenced. Those with no staining of hMSH-2 or hMSH-6 would go straight to gene sequencing (see Fig. 9.1).

Clinical Diagnosis of HNPCC

Following a diagnosis of colorectal cancer, every patient should have a family history taken as part of a complete workup. Potentially all members of a family are at risk. The family history should include three generations with information on colorectal, endometrial, and other HNPCC-associated cancers, and the age of onset of each affected individual. Families that have cancer occurring at a young age, or who demonstrate multiple cancers with vertical transmission from one generation

Table 9.2 Guideline established for clinical recognition of patients at risk for HNPCC

Guidelines	Criteria
Amsterdam 1	1. Three affected family members with histologically proven colorectal cancer, and one must be a first-degree relative of the other two 2. At least two successive generations must be affected 3. At least one family member diagnosed with colorectal cancer prior to age 50 4. Must exclude familial adenomatous polyposis (FAP)
Amsterdam 2	1. At least three relatives with a hereditary non-polyposis colorectal cancer (HNPCC)-associated cancer (colorectal, endometrial, ovarian, gastric, hepatobiliary, small bowel, brain, ureter/renal pelvis, or sebaceous tumors of the skin) 2. One is a first-degree relative of the other two 3. At least two successive generations affected 4. At least one of the HNPCC-associated cancers diagnosed prior to age 50 5. Must exclude FAP in colorectal cancer cases
Original Bethesda (for testing tumors for MSI)	1. Patients with cancer in a family that meets the Amsterdam criteria 2. Patients with two synchronous or metachronous HNPCC-related cancers, including colorectal, endometrial, ovarian, gastric, small bowel, hepatobiliary, brain, ureter/renal pelvis, or sebaceous tumors of the skin 3. Patients with colorectal cancer and a first-degree relative with an HNPCC-associated cancer and/or a colorectal adenoma; one of the cancers must have been diagnosed prior to age 45; the adenoma must have been diagnosed prior to age 40 4. Patients with colorectal or endometrial cancers diagnosed prior to age 45 5. Patients with right-sided colorectal cancer with an undifferentiated histologic pattern (cribriform or solid) diagnosed prior to age 45 6. Patients with a signet ring colorectal carcinoma diagnosed prior to age 45 7. Patients with adenomas diagnosed prior to age 40
Revised Bethesda	1. Colorectal cancer in a patient less than 50 years of age 2. Presence of synchronous or metachronous colorectal or other HNPCC-related tumor at any age 3. Colorectal cancer with typical HNPCC histology (tumor-infiltrating lymphocytes, Crohn's like lymphocytic reaction, mucinous/signet ring cell differentiation, or medullary growth pattern) in a patient less than 60 years of age 4. Colorectal cancer and at least one first-degree relative with an HNPCC-related tumor, with one of the cancers diagnosed at age less than 50 years (or colorectal adenoma diagnosed at age less than 40 years) 5. Two first- or second-degree relatives with HNPCC-related tumors, any age

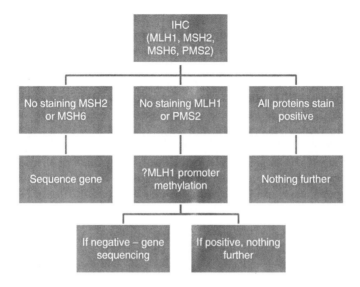

Fig. 9.1 Option for screening all patients with colorectal cancer for HNPCC

to the next and/or with multiple affected relatives, should arouse suspicion of an inherited colorectal cancer syndrome. Once identified, the family should be referred on to a genetic counselor or other qualified individual associated with an inherited cancer registry or inherited cancer clinic [27]. After informed consent of the patient and other family members, all diagnoses are confirmed through patient records, pathology reports or death certificates. Should the family meet the Amsterdam criteria as outlined above they may be offered mismatch repair gene testing.

If tumor tissue is available, the pathologist may test for the common mismatch repair genes with immunohistochemistry or test for microsatellite instability using the Bethesda criteria. While a positive result is suspicious for an MSI tumor, the diagnosis of HNPCC must be confirmed with mismatch repair gene testing. Once a specific genetic mutation is identified, it is relatively easy to test all other family members approximately half of whom will test positive in keeping with its autosomal dominant inheritance pattern. Usually family members are tested around the age they would start screening at 20–25 years or 10 years younger than the youngest affected member in the family.

Screening

Risk of Colorectal Cancer

The risk of colorectal cancer as estimated from high-risk clinics is 70% by 70 years of age with an average age at diagnosis of first cancer in the mid-40s [18, 28], approximately 10 years earlier than sporadic colorectal cancer. This differs from a recent population-based study in which the average age of first HNPCC cancer was 54 years for men and 60 years for women [29]. There is evidence for a differential risk of cancer between the four most commonly mutated genes [20, 30–32]. However, the absolute risk for each gene is unknown at this time. The risk of colorectal cancer is higher in MLH1 mutation carriers than in MSH2 mutation carriers, whereas MSH2 mutation carriers are at higher risk of extracolonic tumors [20, 30, 33]. The risk of colorectal cancer appears to be reduced by one-third in MSH6 mutation carriers compared with that in MLH1 and MSH2 mutation carriers [32, 33]. Whether mutations within a given segment of each specific gene confer greater or lesser risk remains to be determined. Compounding interpretations of these studies are differences in the relative proportion of gene mutations in different ethnic populations and the relatively low incidence of MSH6 and PMS2 mutations; mutations in MLH1 and MSH2 account for approximately 90% of all mutations.

Colonic Surveillance

The goal of surveillance is the early detection of adenomas and asymptomatic cancers. Colorectal cancers arise in HNPCC primarily through the adenoma carcinoma sequence [34]. As a preventative measure, colonoscopic surveillance has been recommended for HNPCC patients since the 1980s. However, the optimal screening interval and age of onset remain unknown.

Overall, patients with HNPCC are at higher risk of adenomas. In a study by Lindgren, the mean age at first observed adenoma was 43 years, with a higher penetrance in men. The relative risk of an adenoma in a patient with HNPCC was 4.5 compared with that in the general population presenting with an adenoma before 54 years of age [35]. The adenoma carcinoma sequence in HNPCC is unique in several respects. Typically, there are fewer than 10 adenomas at first colonoscopy but they are often more advanced [36]. Polyps are larger, and have more dysplastic features including mucinous components and villous architecture. When compared with sporadic cancers, tumor initiation appears to be normal but tumor progression is accelerated [35, 37]. There are a number of well-documented cases of interval colon cancer following a negative colonoscopy [37, 38]. Thus, any decision for surveillance must be accompanied by thorough counseling about HNPCC including its natural history and above all the importance of compliance with surveillance recommendations [39]. In addition, the possibility of missing a small advanced polyp must be considered [40]. HNPCC cancers are often small and flat and can be easily missed during a cursory examination. Patients who are noncompliant or have difficult colonoscopies due to redundancy or fixed angulation should be considered for prophylactic colectomy.

While there are no randomized controlled trials of systematic surveillance in HNPCC, the best available evidence suggests that mutation carriers and patients with clinical criteria suspicious for HNPCC will benefit from an organized screening program. A number of observational studies of surveillance have been published [38, 41–43]. Although of varying quality, all of these studies demonstrate a reduction in colorectal cancer incidence with screening. The observational cohort study by Jarvinen et al. [41] demonstrated a 62% reduction in cancer incidence for patients undergoing colonic screening at 3-year intervals compared with that in individuals from the same families who were unscreened. A follow-up study of this same cohort demonstrated a reduction in mortality from colorectal cancer in those undergoing screening colonoscopy [38]. Cancers that were detected in the screened group were at an early stage and did not lead to death. A study of 114 Dutch families from a national registry with proven or suspected hereditary mismatch repair mutations found that a screening interval of 2 years or less also resulted in the diagnosis of colorectal cancers at an earlier stage [42]. Finally, a prospective observational study from the UK of 554 at-risk persons from 290 families with known mismatch repair gene mutations or families, who fulfilled the Amsterdam criteria, demonstrated a 1% incidence of invasive colorectal cancer and a 5% incidence of high-risk adenomas with a median of 3.3 years between colonoscopies [43]. The reduction in expected mortality was attributed to colonoscopic surveillance.

Despite the methodological limitations of each of these studies, the evidence supports screening for this high-risk population. Based on the available data, a number of guidelines have been published by different interest groups [39, 44–47]. All recommend frequent screening starting at an early age. In general, patients and family members who are known carriers of an HNPCC mutation should undergo lifetime screening with colonoscopy starting at 20–25 years of age with an interval ranging from 1 to 2 years and increasing to annually after age 40. Family members who test negative for a known mutation do not have HNPCC and may be screened using the guidelines for average risk individuals. Families with a clinically suspicious history for HNPCC, where a mutation cannot be identified, must undergo regular screening indefinitely as per the recommendations for HNPCC.

Endometrial Surveillance

Endometrial cancer in HNPCC occurs around 50 years of age, 10 years younger than in the general population [48]. Most patients present with stage I disease with survival rates approaching 90% [48, 49]. Whether screening can improve on this is unknown. In addition, unlike colorectal cancer, there are no screening programs for endometrial cancer in the general population to serve as a baseline for comparison. Women with HNPCC who are at risk of endometrial cancer are younger and more likely to be premenopausal. Abnormal bleeding may not be recognized as such and thus some form of screening seems appropriate [44].

Suggested methods of endometrial screening include endometrial sampling and transvaginal ultrasound. Studies of transvaginal ultrasound measuring the endometrial thickness have demonstrated a high false-positive rate when used in high-risk populations [50, 51]. However, transvaginal ultrasound may also be useful in examining the ovaries. Endometrial biopsy has not been investigated as a screening tool in this population. Despite the limited evidence, most guidelines suggest transvaginal ultrasound and aspiration biopsy of the endometrium starting at 30–35 years with an interval ranging from 1 to 2 years.

Screening for Other Cancers

Although cancers other than endometrial or colorectal collectively comprise about 30% of the cancers seen in MLH1/MSH2 families, and possibly 50% of the cancers in MSH6 families, there is no evidence that screening for these cancers will improve survival [33]. Most authors recommend screening only for families with a strong history of the cancer in question. HNPCC families from countries such as China and Korea, where gastric cancer is endemic in the general population, also seem to be at higher risk of gastric cancer [52–54].

Prophylactic Surgery

Colectomy

There is no evidence for or against prophylactic colectomy in Lynch syndrome and in contrast to FAP prophylactic colectomy is rarely performed. This is due in part to the variable penetrance of the disease. Most families demonstrate a 60–80% penetrance, thus as many as 40% of patients would undergo unnecessary surgery. On the other hand, families with close to 100% penetrance may choose this option as colonoscopic surveillance is not 100% guaranteed to prevent colorectal cancer [55, 56]. In a decision analysis, Syngal compared surveillance to prophylactic subtotal colectomy [57]. Although both colonoscopic surveillance and prophylactic surgery led to big gains in life expectancy, the benefits of colectomy over colonoscopy decreased with advancing age. Thus the decision must be individualized and based on family risk, patient preference, adherence to screening guidelines, and ease of screening. In general, a subtotal colectomy is the procedure of choice with lifelong surveillance of the rectal remnant.

Hysterectomy and Oophorectomy

Women with Lynch syndrome must decide between screening and prophylactic surgery given the increased risk for endometrial cancer and ovarian cancer. Families with an MSH6 mutation have the highest risk of developing endometrial cancer. While there are no data regarding screening, there is evidence for the benefits of prophylactic surgery [58]. Schmeler reported on a retrospective cohort of 315 women with an MSI mutation, 61 of whom had a prophylactic hysterectomy and bilateral oophorectomy. At 10 years of follow up, no endometrial or ovarian cancer developed in those who had prophylactic surgery whereas 33% of those who did not have surgery developed endometrial cancer and 5.5% developed ovarian cancer. Based on these data, a prophylactic hysterectomy and bilateral oophorectomy is a reasonable option and should be considered for HNPCC patients who are post menopausal or when child bearing is complete. There is no evidence at present that this strategy will affect overall survival. Thus, a complete discussion of the risks, benefits, and alternatives is required. There are no specific contraindications to hormone replacement therapy in patients with HNPCC [44].

Other Cancers

There is no evidence for or against prophylactic surgery for any other HNPCC-associated cancers.

Colorectal Cancer Treatment

There are no randomized controlled trials comparing segmental colectomy with subtotal colectomy for patients with Lynch syndrome who develop colorectal cancer. One decision analysis has concluded an increased life expectancy with subtotal colectomy compared with partial resection but no one operation is best for all patients. Considerations include patient compliance, baseline bowel function (preoperative frequency or loose stools), impaired sphincter function, age, ease of colonoscopy, and patient's wishes.

Colon Cancer

Approximately 60–70% of colon cancers in Lynch syndrome are proximal to the splenic flexure [59]. When considering operative treatment, there are two primary goals: first, resection of the primary lesion with appropriate margins and optimal lymph node sampling; and second, reduction of the remaining at-risk mucosa. There are three operative choices including a right hemicolectomy, an extended right hemicolectomy, and a total abdominal colectomy with an ileorectal anastomosis. Most patients will be offered total abdominal colectomy. In addition to treating the primary cancer, it eliminates most of the at-risk mucosa thereby reducing the lifetime risk of metachronous cancers which may be as high as 40% within 7 years of the first primary [20]. In addition, it preserves anal/sphincter function, retains the reservoir function of the rectum and eliminates the need for surveillance colonoscopy. Surveillance of the rectum is required as the estimated risk of cancer in the retained rectum is 12% at 12 years [60]. A simple right hemicolectomy or extended right hemicolectomy may be considered when operative risks including comorbidities, age or borderline continence outweigh future cancer risk [47]. Left colon cancer is much rarer. These lesions may be treated with a total abdominal colectomy and ileorectal anastomosis or by formal left hemicolectomy based on similar considerations.

Rectal Cancer

Rectal cancer is uncommon in Lynch syndrome. Accepted procedures for cancers not involving the sphincters include an anterior proctosigmoidectomy with colorectal or coloanal anastomosis and a total proctocolectomy with or without an ileoanal pouch. As with colon cancer, the choice of procedure must be individualized; bowel function and continence become an important factor. Rectal cancers should be staged with endorectal ultrasound and/or MRI. In locally advanced cancers, chemoradiation should be given preoperatively. If an ileal pouch is being considered in this setting, chemoradiation should be given prior to pouch construction as the pouch tolerates radiation very poorly. Decisions regarding the need for an abdomino-perineal resection are based on the same criteria as for sporadic tumors. In general, if sphincter preservation is not possible, a proctocolectomy and end ileostomy should be considered to eliminate the remaining at-risk mucosa.

Adenomas

While most adenomas can be removed endoscopically, some due to size or location require surgical resection. Other polyps are small and flat and may be unsuitable for endoscopic removal. Again the extent of resection should be determined primarily by patient preference, compliance with screening, ease of screening, and polyp location. The surgical options are the same as those for cancers. Occasionally, patients present with multiple adenomas in isolation or in combination with a cancer where a more extensive resection is indicated.

Outcomes

Survival

Overall survival rates for HNPCC in retrospective studies are better than that of patients with sporadic colorectal cancer, with a reported 10-year survival of 69%

vs. 48% in sporadic cancer [18]. This difference persists when patients are matched stage for stage and for age of onset [22, 61]. Stage II patients with transmural penetration, stage III patients, and stage IV patients all have fewer distant metastasis than expected when compared with sporadic tumors. It has been postulated that this increased survival is due to heightened immune surveillance. Tumor infiltrating lymphocytes that are seen on pathologic examination are felt to be associated with a host immune response although the exact mechanism of action is unknown. In contrast, Barnetson et al. recently examined survival in a large population-based study of colorectal cancer patients, comparing HNPCC carriers with noncarriers. There was no significant difference in survival between carriers and noncarriers with a reported 5-year survival of 74% and 63%, respectively [62]. In addition, when compared stage for stage, there was no survival difference. This study has been criticized for the low number of carriers present in the population. Additional prospective research is needed to fully answer this question.

Chemotherapy

At the present time, there are three chemotherapeutic agents with proven effectiveness in colorectal cancer: 5-FU with or without leucovorin, oxaliplatin, and irinotecan. Although the effectiveness of these agents in MSI tumors or patients with Lynch syndrome is unknown, there is evidence to suggest that MSI-H tumors are resistant to 5-FU-based chemotherapy in vitro [63]. There are very few studies that address this question clinically. Three retrospective studies [64–66] demonstrated no difference in survival between patients with MSI-H tumors who received 5-FU chemotherapy and those who did not. The study by Ribic was novel in that tissue specimens were obtained from patients previously enrolled in randomized controlled trials of fluorouracil-based chemotherapy where patients were prospectively followed and the outcome known. As expected, in the group of patients who did not receive adjuvant chemotherapy those with high-frequency microsatellite unstable tumors demonstrated an increase in survival when compared with patients with low-frequency microsatellite unstable or microsatellite stable tumors. Among patients who received adjuvant chemotherapy, those with microsatellite stable or low frequency unstable tumors demonstrated an increase in survival whereas patients with high-frequency microsatellite unstable tumors did not benefit from adjuvant chemotherapy [64].

A single nonrandomized study of stage IV patients demonstrated better survival in MSI-H patients who received 5-FU-based chemotherapy [67]. This difference could be due to the underlying cause of the MSI; germline mutations in HNPCC vs. MLH1 promoter gene methylation in sporadic MSI tumors. A single study of irinotecan in stage IV patients reported complete or partial response to irinotecan in four of seven patients. As these studies are either retrospective or small, no definitive conclusions can be drawn. Specific recommendations await confirmation with prospective clinical trials.

References

1. Warthin AS. Heredity with reference to carcinomas as shown by the case study of the cases examined in the pathological laboratory of the University of Michigan, 1895–1913. Arch Intern Med 1913; 12:546–555.
2. Lynch HT, Shaw MW, Magnuson CW, et al. Hereditary factors in cancer. Study of two large midwestern kindreds. Arch Intern Med 1966; 117:206–212.
3. Lynch HT, Krush AJ. The cancer family syndrome and cancer control. Surg Gynecol Obstet 1971; 132:247–250.
4. Lynch HT, Harris RE, Organ CH, Jr., et al. The surgeon, genetics, and cancer control: the Cancer Family Syndrome. Ann Surg 1977; 185:435–440.
5. Vasen HF, Mecklin JP, Khan PM, Lynch HT. The International Collaborative Group on Hereditary Non-Polyposis Colorectal Cancer (ICG-HNPCC). Dis Colon Rectum 1991; 34:424–425.
6. Rodriguez-Bigas MA, Boland CR, Hamilton SR, et al. A National Cancer Institute Workshop on Hereditary Nonpolyposis Colorectal Cancer Syndrome: meeting highlights and Bethesda guidelines. J Natl Cancer Inst 1997; 89:1758–1762.
7. Vasen HF, Watson P, Mecklin JP, Lynch HT. New clinical criteria for hereditary nonpolyposis colorectal cancer (HNPCC, Lynch syndrome) proposed by the International Collaborative group on HNPCC. Gastroenterology 1999; 116:1453–1456.
8. Aaltonen LA, Peltomaki P. Genes involved in hereditary nonpolyposis colorectal carcinoma. Anticancer Res 1994; 14:1657–1660.
9. Peltomaki P, Aaltonen LA, Sistonen P, et al. Genetic mapping of a locus predisposing to human colorectal cancer. Science 1993; 260:810–812.
10. Lindblom A, Tannergard P, Werelius B, Nordenskjold M. Genetic mapping of a second locus predisposing to hereditary non-polyposis colon cancer. Nat Genet 1993; 5:279–282.
11. Leach FS, Nicolaides NC, Papadopoulos N, et al. Mutations of a mutS homolog in hereditary nonpolyposis colorectal cancer. Cell 1993; 75:1215–1225.
12. Bronner CE, Baker SM, Morrison PT, et al. Mutation in the DNA mismatch repair gene homologue hMLH1 is associated with hereditary non-polyposis colon cancer. Nature 1994; 368:258–261.
13. Papadopoulos N, Nicolaides NC, Wei YF, et al. Mutation of a mutL homolog in hereditary colon cancer. Science 1994; 263:1625–1629.
14. Miyaki M, Konishi M, Tanaka K, et al. Germline mutation of MSH6 as the cause of hereditary nonpolyposis colorectal cancer. Nat Genet 1997; 17:271–272.
15. Nicolaides NC, Papadopoulos N, Liu B, et al. Mutations of two PMS homologues in hereditary nonpolyposis colon cancer. Nature 1994; 371:75–80.
16. Akiyama Y, Tsubouchi N, Yuasa Y. Frequent somatic mutations of hMSH3 with reference to microsatellite instability in hereditary nonpolyposis colorectal cancers. Biochem Biophys Res Commun 1997; 236:248–252.
17. Jackson-Thompson J, Ahmed F, German RR, et al. Descriptive epidemiology of colorectal cancer in the United States, 1998–2001. Cancer 2006; 107:1103–1111.
18. Lynch HT, de la Chapelle A. Hereditary colorectal cancer. N Engl J Med 2003; 348:919–932.
19. Rodriguez-Bigas MA, Chang GJ, Skibber JM. Surgical implications of colorectal cancer genetics. Surg Oncol Clin N Am 2006; 15:51–66, vi.
20. Lin KM, Shashidharan M, Ternent CA, et al. Colorectal and extracolonic cancer variations in MLH1/MSH2 hereditary nonpolyposis colorectal cancer kindreds and the general population. Dis Colon Rectum 1998; 41:428–433.
21. Brown SR, Finan PJ, Hall NR, Bishop DT. Incidence of DNA replication errors in patients with multiple primary cancers. Dis Colon Rectum 1998; 41:765–769.
22. Watson P, Lin KM, Rodriguez-Bigas MA, et al. Colorectal carcinoma survival among hereditary nonpolyposis colorectal carcinoma family members. Cancer 1998; 83:259–266.

23. Bandipalliam P. Syndrome of early onset colon cancers, hematologic malignancies & features of neurofibromatosis in HNPCC families with homozygous mismatch repair gene mutations. Fam Cancer 2005; 4:323–333.
24. Syngal S, Fox EA, Eng C, et al. Sensitivity and specificity of clinical criteria for hereditary non-polyposis colorectal cancer associated mutations in MSH2 and MLH1. J Med Genet 2000; 37:641–645.
25. Wolf B, Gruber S, Henglmueller S, et al. Efficiency of the revised Bethesda guidelines (2003) for the detection of mutations in mismatch repair genes in Austrian HNPCC patients. Int J Cancer 2006; 118:1465–1470.
26. Hampel H, Frankel WL, Martin E, et al. Screening for the Lynch syndrome (hereditary non-polyposis colorectal cancer). N Engl J Med 2005; 352:1851–1860.
27. Church JM, Kay S, Shenae J. The benefits of genetic counselling in families likely to have HNPCC and why families do not get it. Dis Colon Rectum 2005; 48:616 [Generic].
28. Gruber SB. New developments in Lynch syndrome (hereditary nonpolyposis colorectal cancer) and mismatch repair gene testing. Gastroenterology 2006; 130:577–587.
29. Hampel H, Stephens JA, Pukkala E, et al. Cancer risk in hereditary nonpolyposis colorectal cancer syndrome: later age of onset. Gastroenterology 2005; 129:415–421.
30. Vasen HF, Wijnen JT, Menko FH, et al. Cancer risk in families with hereditary nonpolyposis colorectal cancer diagnosed by mutation analysis. Gastroenterology 1996; 110:1020–1027.
31. Nakagawa H, Lockman JC, Frankel WL, et al. Mismatch repair gene PMS2: disease-causing germline mutations are frequent in patients whose tumors stain negative for PMS2 protein, but paralogous genes obscure mutation detection and interpretation. Cancer Res 2004; 64:4721–4727.
32. Hendriks YM, Wagner A, Morreau H, et al. Cancer risk in hereditary nonpolyposis colorectal cancer due to MSH6 mutations: impact on counseling and surveillance. Gastroenterology 2004; 127:17–25.
33. Plaschke J, Engel C, Kruger S, et al. Lower incidence of colorectal cancer and later age of disease onset in 27 families with pathogenic MSH6 germline mutations compared with families with MLH1 or MSH2 mutations: the German Hereditary Nonpolyposis Colorectal Cancer Consortium. J Clin Oncol 2004; 22:4486–4494.
34. Mecklin JP, Aarnio M, Laara E, et al. Development of colorectal tumors in colonoscopic surveillance in Lynch syndrome. Gastroenterology 2007; 133:1093–1098.
35. Lindgren G, Liljegren A, Jaramillo E, et al. Adenoma prevalence and cancer risk in familial non-polyposis colorectal cancer. Gut 2002; 50:228–234.
36. Jass JR. Colorectal adenomas in surgical specimens from subjects with hereditary non-polyposis colorectal cancer. Histopathology 1995; 27:263–267.
37. Vasen HF, Taal BG, Nagengast FM, et al. Hereditary nonpolyposis colorectal cancer: results of long-term surveillance in 50 families. Eur J Cancer 1995; 31A:1145–1148.
38. Jarvinen HJ, Aarnio M, Mustonen H, et al. Controlled 15-year trial on screening for colorectal cancer in families with hereditary nonpolyposis colorectal cancer. Gastroenterology 2000; 118:829–834.
39. Church J, Simmang C et al. Practice parameters for the treatment of patients with dominantly inherited colorectal cancer (familial adenomatous polyposis and hereditary nonpolyposis colorectal cancer). Dis Colon Rectum 2003; 46:1001–1012.
40. Rex DK, Cutler CS, Lemmel GT, et al. Colonoscopic miss rates of adenomas determined by back-to-back colonoscopies. Gastroenterology 1997; 112:24–28.
41. Jarvinen HJ, Mecklin JP, Sistonen P. Screening reduces colorectal cancer rate in families with hereditary nonpolyposis colorectal cancer. Gastroenterology 1995; 108:1405–1411.
42. de Vos tot Nederveen Cappel WH, Nagengast FM, Griffioen G, et al. Surveillance for hereditary nonpolyposis colorectal cancer: a long-term study on 114 families. Dis Colon Rectum 2002; 45:1588–1594.
43. Dove-Edwin I, Sasieni P, Adams J, Thomas HJ. Prevention of colorectal cancer by colonoscopic surveillance in individuals with a family history of colorectal cancer: 16 year, prospective, follow-up study. BMJ 2005; 331:1047.

44. Lindor NM, Petersen GM, Hadley DW, et al. Recommendations for the care of individuals with an inherited predisposition to Lynch syndrome: a systematic review. JAMA 2006; 296:1507–1517.
45. National Comprehensive Care Network. NCCN practice guidelines in oncology. Colorectal Cancer Screening V.I.2007. http://www.nccn.org/professionals/physician_gls/PDF/colorectal_screening.pdf. 2007.
46. Levin B, Lieberman DA, McFarland B, et al. Screening and Surveillance for the Early Detection of Colorectal Cancer and Adenomatous Polyps, 2008: A Joint Guideline from the American Cancer Society, the US Multi-Society Task Force on Colorectal Cancer, and the American College of Radiology. CA Cancer J Clin 2008:LS1.
47. Vasen HF, Moslein G, Alonso A, et al. Guidelines for the clinical management of Lynch syndrome (hereditary non-polyposis cancer). J Med Genet 2007; 44:353–362.
48. Broaddus RR, Lynch HT, Chen LM, et al. Pathologic features of endometrial carcinoma associated with HNPCC: a comparison with sporadic endometrial carcinoma. Cancer 2006; 106:87–94.
49. Boks DE, Trujillo AP, Voogd AC, et al. Survival analysis of endometrial carcinoma associated with hereditary nonpolyposis colorectal cancer. Int J Cancer 2002; 102:198–200.
50. Rijcken FE, Mourits MJ, Kleibeuker JH, et al. Gynecologic screening in hereditary nonpolyposis colorectal cancer. Gynecol Oncol 2003; 91:74–80.
51. Dove-Edwin I, Boks D, Goff S, et al. The outcome of endometrial carcinoma surveillance by ultrasound scan in women at risk of hereditary nonpolyposis colorectal carcinoma and familial colorectal carcinoma. Cancer 2002; 94:1708–1712.
52. Park YJ, Shin KH, Park JG. Risk of gastric cancer in hereditary nonpolyposis colorectal cancer in Korea. Clin Cancer Res 2000; 6:2994–2998.
53. Zhang YZ, Sheng JQ, Li SR, Zhang H. Clinical phenotype and prevalence of hereditary nonpolyposis colorectal cancer syndrome in Chinese population. World J Gastroenterol 2005; 11:1481–1488.
54. Liu SR, Zhao B, Wang ZJ, et al. Clinical features and mismatch repair gene mutation screening in Chinese patients with hereditary nonpolyposis colorectal carcinoma. World J Gastroenterol 2004; 10:2647–2651.
55. Corleto VD, Zykaj E, Mercantini P, et al. Is colonoscopy sufficient for colorectal cancer surveillance in all HNPCC patients? World J Gastroenterol 2005; 11:7541–7544.
56. Church J. Hereditary colon cancers can be tiny: a cautionary case report of the results of colonoscopic surveillance. Am J Gastroenterol 1998; 93:2289–2290.
57. Syngal S, Weeks JC, Schrag D, et al. Benefits of colonoscopic surveillance and prophylactic colectomy in patients with hereditary nonpolyposis colorectal cancer mutations. Ann Intern Med 1998; 129:787–796.
58. Schmeler KM, Lynch HT, Chen LM, et al. Prophylactic surgery to reduce the risk of gynecologic cancers in the Lynch syndrome. N Engl J Med 2006; 354:261–269.
59. Lynch HT, Watson P, Lanspa SJ, et al. Natural history of colorectal cancer in hereditary nonpolyposis colorectal cancer (Lynch syndromes I and II). Dis Colon Rectum 1988; 31:439–444.
60. Rodriguez-Bigas MA, Vasen HF, Pekka-Mecklin J, et al. Rectal cancer risk in hereditary nonpolyposis colorectal cancer after abdominal colectomy. International Collaborative Group on HNPCC. Ann Surg 1997; 225:202–207.
61. Sankila R, Aaltonen LA, Jarvinen HJ, Mecklin JP. Better survival rates in patients with MLH1-associated hereditary colorectal cancer. Gastroenterology 1996; 110:682–687.
62. Barnetson RA, Tenesa A, Farrington SM, et al. Identification and survival of carriers of mutations in DNA mismatch-repair genes in colon cancer. N Engl J Med 2006; 354:2751–2763.
63. Carethers JM, Chauhan DP, Fink D, et al. Mismatch repair proficiency and in vitro response to 5-fluorouracil. Gastroenterology 1999; 117:123–131.
64. Ribic CM, Sargent DJ, Moore MJ, et al. Tumor microsatellite-instability status as a predictor of benefit from fluorouracil-based adjuvant chemotherapy for colon cancer. N Engl J Med 2003; 349:247–257.

65. Carethers JM, Smith EJ, Behling CA, et al. Use of 5-fluorouracil and survival in patients with microsatellite-unstable colorectal cancer. Gastroenterology 2004; 126:394–401.
66. de Vos tot Nederveen Cappel WH, Meulenbeld HJ, Kleibeuker JH, et al. Survival after adjuvant 5-FU treatment for stage III colon cancer in hereditary nonpolyposis colorectal cancer. Int J Cancer 2004; 109:468–471.
67. Liang JT, Huang KC, Lai HS, et al. High-frequency microsatellite instability predicts better chemosensitivity to high-dose 5-fluorouracil plus leucovorin chemotherapy for stage IV sporadic colorectal cancer after palliative bowel resection. Int J Cancer 2002; 101:519–525.

Chapter 10
Hereditary Ovarian Cancer and Other Gynecologic Malignancies

Kathryn R. Brown and Lynn P. Parker

Although the majority of gynecologic malignancies are sporadic, there is a subset of patients who develop genetic forms of gynecologic cancer. Advances in molecular biology have allowed for an understanding of the physiological pathways of development of inherited gynecologic malignancies and the identification of genetic alterations that lead to the malignant phenotype. The aim of this chapter is to help the clinician identify those patients who are at risk for developing inherited forms of gynecologic malignancies and who would benefit from screening, chemoprevention, and surgery.

Ovarian Carcinoma

Genetic Abnormalities in High-Risk Individuals

Modern molecular biology techniques have allowed identification of associated genetic mutations in ovarian cancer. Research by Easton et al. identified a genetic link between ovarian cancer and mutations in the *BRCA1* gene [1]. Initial research linking *BRCA1* and *BRCA2* to elevated risk of ovarian cancer suggested a cumulative risk of ovarian cancer of 63% by age 70, where the normal population risk approximates 1.6% [1]. A higher frequency of ovarian cancer and associated *BRCA* mutations has also been shown in women of Ashkenazi Jewish descent further supporting the belief that the elevated risk of ovarian cancer is an inherited phenomenon [2]. Subsequent studies expanded the patient population with associated *BRCA1* and *BRCA2* mutations resulting in a reduction in the estimated lifetime risk of ovarian cancer in these patients. Based on the analysis of multiple studies, the average cumulative risk of ovarian cancer is 39% in *BRCA1* mutation carriers

K.R. Brown (✉)
Department of Obstetrics, Gynecology and Women's Health, University of Louisville Hospital, Louisville, KY 40202, USA
e-mail: krbrown14@gwise.louisville.edu

C.N. Ellis (ed.), *Inherited Cancer Syndromes: Current Clinical Management*,
DOI 10.1007/978-1-4419-6821-0_10, © Springer Science+Business Media, LLC 2011

and 11% in *BRCA2* mutation carriers [3]. Although the risk of ovarian cancer is lower in *BRCA2* mutation carriers, the high susceptibility observed in the risk of breast cancer persists [4].

Multiple studies of patients with family histories suggestive of an increased risk of familial ovarian cancer reported the *BRCA* gene to be mutated in 0–50% of patients [5–7]. Sutcliffe et al., using the UKCCCR Cancer registry, retrospectively identified patients having two or more first-degree relatives diagnosed with ovarian cancer [8]. In this patient cohort, a relative risk of developing ovarian cancer remained elevated at 11–59% when no abnormality in *BRCA1* was noted. A Gynecologic Oncology Group study prospectively identified ovarian cancer patients with significant family histories of breast and ovarian cancer [7]. Of 26 eligible patients screened for mutations, 46% (12) had abnormalities in the *BRCA* genes (*BRCA1–8* mutations and *BRCA2–4* mutations). An increasing frequency of these mutations was observed as the number of affected relatives increased.

While population-based studies establish a link between mutations in the *BRCA1* gene and a risk of ovarian cancer, laboratory studies suggest an actual role for the *BRCA* gene as a tumor suppressor [9]. The *BRCA1* and *BRCA2* genes encode proteins involved in repair of double-stranded DNA breaks by homologous recombination [10]. Defects in these genes prevent the repair of the double-stranded DNA breaks resulting in chromosomal abnormalities and genetic instability. Transcriptional regulation of the p53 and p21 promoters and alteration of Rad51 protein, which localizes the double-stranded DNA breaks, appear to be influenced by the *BRCA* protein product [11, 12]. This inability to repair the double-stranded DNA breaks theoretically may make patients with *BRCA* mutations very sensitive to platinum chemotherapy, which works by this same mechanism.

The mechanism of development of *BRCA*-associated ovarian cancer is hypothesized to arise from ovarian surface epithelium (OSE) (Fig. 10.1). Following ovulation, the OSE proliferates and may become internalized in inclusion cysts. The OSE is exposed to growth factors and hormones within the ovarian stroma and continues to proliferate. Mutations that subsequently occur cannot be repaired due to the *BRCA* mutation. The uncontrolled cellular growth eventually leads to cancer [13].

Multiple etiologies of ovarian cancer can and do exist; therefore, not all inherited forms of epithelial ovarian cancer are attributable to *BRCA1* and *BRCA2* mutations. Stratton et al. suggested that *BRCA1* mutations occur in only 5% of sporadic ovarian cancers observed in patients less than age 70 [14]. These other genetic mutations encompass alterations in both known and unknown ovarian cancer genes, an important concept when counseling patients regarding inherited risk. When a defined *BRCA* mutation is present in a pedigree affected by multiple cases of breast and ovarian cancer, either a positive or negative test may be useful in clinical decision making. However, if the *BRCA* gene is normal through multiple affected relatives, then the contributed risk may be due to other inheritable genetic alterations making *BRCA* testing less helpful.

Hereditary nonpolyposis colorectal cancer (HNPCC), or Lynch syndrome, is an autosomal-dominant genetic syndrome where an elevated risk of ovarian cancer is observed. HNPCC is associated with germline mutations in the *MLH1*, *MSH2*, *MSH6*, and *PMS2* genes resulting in defects of DNA mismatch repair leading to

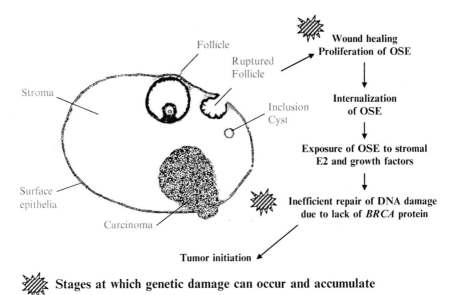

Follicle

Ruptured
Follicle

Stroma

Inclusion
Cyst

Surface
epithelia

Carcinoma

Wound healing
Proliferation of OSE

Internalization
of OSE

Exposure of OSE to stromal
E2 and growth factors

Inefficient repair of DNA damage
due to lack of *BRCA* protein

Tumor initiation

Stages at which genetic damage can occur and accumulate

Fig. 10.1 Development of ovarian cancer in *BRCA* mutation carriers. The OSE is a single layer of cells contiguous with the peritoneal mesothelium. Even in the normal surface context OSE cells have a more differentiated phenotype than peritoneal cells, presumably due to their proximity to the hormones and growth factors produced by the ovarian stroma and follicles. Ovulation results in the instigation of wound healing and OSE proliferation to repair the membrane ruptured during the release of the follicle. Invaginations of the OSE occur during the repair process, and with repeated ovulation these can be internalized to form inclusion cysts. It is thought that these inclusion cysts are fertile environments for ovarian carcinoma development, due to their exposure to the ovarian stroma. Women with a mutation in *BRCA1* or *BRCA2* are less able to cope with DNA damage inflicted on the cells and accumulate mutations during proliferation and estrogen exposure, leading to the initiation of an epithelial tumor (from HM Sowter and A Ashworth [13], by permission of Oxford University Press)

microsatellite instability [15]. Cohort studies document the lifetime risk of ovarian cancer in female patients with HNPCC is approximately 13% [16]. Furthermore, ovarian cancer occurs in 2% of patients with HNPCC-associated mutations [17].

The majority of ovarian cancers detected in *BRCA* mutation carriers tend to be invasive serous carcinomas with a statistically significant higher histologic grade [18]. However, rare ovarian tumor types associated with uncommon genetic syndromes have been reported. Ollier's disease is associated with the development of juvenile granulosa cell tumors [19]. Approximately one-third of patients diagnosed with ovarian sex cord tumors with annular tubules have Peutz–Jeghers syndrome [20]. Gorlin's syndrome is associated with an inherited predisposition to develop benign ovarian fibromas [21]. Patients with ataxia telangiectasia, an autosomal-recessive disorder with a gene abnormality identified on chromosome 11q, have been reported to develop ovarian dysgerminoma [22]. Gonadoblastoma, a tumor with both germ cell and sex cord stromal elements, has been known to develop in patients where a Y chromosome is present, but a female phenotype exists [23]. Patients with gonadoblastoma are predisposed to develop germ cell tumors.

Assessment of Individuals at Elevated Inherited Risk of Ovarian Cancer

Evaluation of a patient who might be considered at elevated risk for ovarian cancer should be initiated in the context of a careful pedigree analysis. Special emphasis should be placed within the pedigree analysis on multiplicity of breast and ovarian cancer within a familial cohort, as well as young age of onset. The National Comprehensive Cancer Network (NCCN) Clinical Practice Guidelines in Oncology details the assessment of high-risk individuals. The NCCN criteria for genetic testing are listed in Table 10.1 [24]. The clinician should recognize that genetic testing encompasses relatively few genes known to place individuals

Table 10.1 NCCN hereditary breast and/or ovarian cancer testing criteria

1. Member of the family with a known *BRCA1/BRCA2* mutation
2. Personal history of breast cancer with one or more of the following:
   - Diagnosed at age ≤45 years, with or without family history
   - Diagnosed at age ≤50 years, with ≥1 close blood relative with breast cancer aged ≤50 years and/or ≥1 close blood relative with epithelial ovarian, fallopian, or primary peritoneal cancer
   - Two breast primaries when first breast cancer diagnosis occurred prior to age 50
   - Diagnosed at any age with ≥2 close blood relatives with breast and/or epithelial ovarian, fallopian, or primary peritoneal cancer at any age
   - Close male blood relative with breast cancer
   - Personal history of epithelial ovarian, fallopian tube, or primary peritoneal cancer
   - For individuals of ethnicity associated with higher mutation frequency (e.g. founder populations of Ashkenazi Jewish, Icelandic, Swedish, Hungarian, or other) no family history may be required, although testing for founder-specific mutations, if available, should be performed first
3. Personal history of epithelial ovarian, fallopian tube, or primary peritoneal cancer
4. Personal history of male breast cancer
5. Family history only – close family member meeting any of the above criteria

Source: Adapted with permission from The NCCN 1.2009 Genetic/Familial High-Risk Assessment: Breast and Ovarian Clinical Practice Guidelines in Oncology. ©National Comprehensive Cancer Network, 2010. Available at: http://www.nccn.org. Accessed January 31, 2010. To view the most recent and complete version of the guideline, go online to www.nccn.org (These guidelines are a work in progress that will be refined as often as new significant data becomes available. The NCCN guidelines are a statement of consensus of its authors regarding their views of current accepted approaches to treatment. Any clinician seeking to apply or consult any NCCN guideline is expected to use independent medical judgment in the context of individual clinical circumstances to determine any patient's care or treatment. The National Comprehensive Cancer Network makes no warranties of any kind whatsoever regarding their content, use or application and disclaims any responsibility for their application or use in any way. These guidelines are copyrighted by the National Comprehensive Cancer Network. All rights reserved. These guidelines and illustrations herein may not be reproduced in any form for any purpose without the express written permission of the NCCN)

at increased risk. Therefore, situations may exist where family history alone is sufficient for considering either a screening or preventative intervention.

While guidelines can help suggest a patient at risk, the decision to perform a genetic test is multifaceted and best determined using a comprehensive multidisciplinary genetic counseling program. Consideration should be given to how the information will be used by the patient and provider, who will receive the results, and how the information will be dispersed throughout the family. The decision process for clinical management of a high-risk patient is outlined in Fig. 10.2. The most useful individual to test is an affected relative, as a test indicating a mutation for *BRCA1/BRCA2* will be more informative than a negative test. A negative test in affected individuals is problematic as other unknown genes may be operative in individual families and mutations may be present in the *BRCA* genes that cannot be identified using current methods. The family risk may also be due to multiple low penetrance genes or the clustering of genes in the family altered by shared environmental risk factors [25]. Therefore, consideration of interventions based on a strong family history alone remains reasonable.

Screening Interventions in High-Risk Individuals

Focus has been placed on screening to identify early stage disease amenable to curative resection since therapeutic intervention of any advanced-stage solid tumor is unlikely to produce a substantial cure rate. The challenge faced with screening interventions is the relatively low prevalence of the disease. Effectiveness of any screening strategy will thus be hindered by a low positive predictive value (PPV). Given an estimated prevalence of 50 cases per 100,000, a test with 99% specificity and 100% sensitivity would yield only one in 21 women undergoing surgical intervention with ovarian cancer [26]. The screening trials performed to date in average risk women would support these problematic statistics. A representative study utilizing screening with both CA125 and ultrasound in 22,000 subjects identified 41 women with positive screening results. Of these 41 women, 11 were noted to have cancer with 70% of these cancers stage III or IV [27]. During screening of 863 CA125 values, 39 were found to be elevated with an overall sensitivity, specificity, and PPV of 50, 96, and 13%, respectively [28].

Studies utilizing screening with CA125 reported substantial numbers of patients with longitudinal CA125 values [27, 29]. Graphical analysis of data suggested that information that differentiates ovarian cancer cases prior to clinical symptoms from all other women was contained in the pattern of CA125 over time [30]. In women subsequently diagnosed with ovarian cancer, CA125 values rose exponentially over time, whereas in most other women CA125 values remained relatively stable over time even when initially elevated. This information is in addition to the traditional interpretation of the CA125 value, whether it exceeds a specified cutoff of 30 or 35 U/mL. Skates et al. addressed the dilemma of low PPV using statistical models of

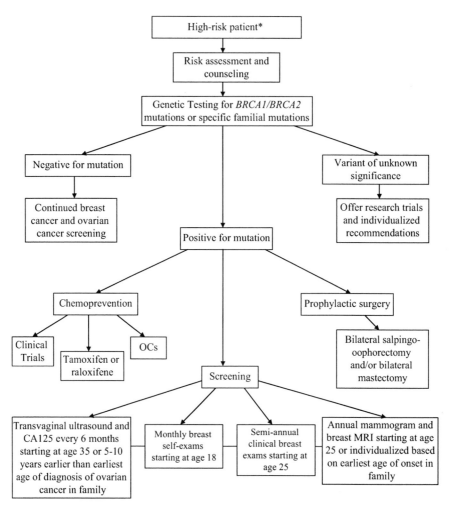

*High-risk patient is defined as a patient meeting NCCN Hereditary Breast and/or Ovarian Cancer testing criteria.

Fig. 10.2 The screening information in this table has been adapted with permission from The NCCN 1.2009 Genetic/Familial High-Risk Assessment: Breast and Ovarian Clinical Practice Guidelines in Oncology. ©National Comprehensive Cancer Network, 2010. Available at: http://www.nccn.org. Accessed January 31, 2010. To view the most recent and complete version of the guideline, go online to www.nccn.org (These guidelines are a work in progress that will be refined as often as new significant data becomes available. The NCCN guidelines are a statement of consensus of its authors regarding their views of current accepted approaches to treatment. Any clinician seeking to apply or consult any NCCN guideline is expected to use independent medical judgment in the context of individual clinical circumstances to determine any patient's care or treatment. The National Comprehensive Cancer Network makes no warranties of any kind whatsoever regarding their content, use, or application and disclaims any responsibility for their application or use in any way. These guidelines are copyrighted by the National Comprehensive Cancer Network. All rights reserved. These guidelines and illustrations herein may not be reproduced in any form for any purpose without the express written permission of the NCCN)

longitudinal CA125 behavior in cases and controls. A method for calculating the probability of ovarian cancer given the subject's CA125 value and age was developed, and this risk of ovarian cancer algorithm (ROCA) efficiently identifies women at higher risk of ovarian cancer for more aggressive interventions. Analysis of the UK and Swedish data demonstrates the power of ROCA with a vast increase in the PPV from 2 to 16% while maintaining a high level of sensitivity of over 80%. The increase in PPV was achieved by using longitudinal information rather than a fixed cutpoint across all subjects [30]. A prospective pilot study using this algorithm in over 13,000 postmenopausal women has confirmed an increased PPV of 19% [31]. The ROCA is also being evaluated in a large UK randomized control trial of ovarian cancer screening.

As a result of the lack of specificity of using CA125 as a screening marker, alternative strategies were developed. Van Nagell et al. have approximated a 10% PPV utilizing an ultrasound screening protocol [32]. In this study, screening ultrasounds were performed on 14,469 "normal risk" women. A total of 17 cancers were identified, of which 11 were stage I, yielding a PPV of 9.4%. A criticism of this study, however, noted that 6 of 11 of the stage I tumors were of a granulosa cell/stromal histology or ovarian tumors of low malignant potential. A similar finding was observed in an ultrasound study by Sato et al. involving 51,550 subjects [33]. Twenty-four tumors were identified, of which 17 were stage I, with 5 of the 17 identified as granulosa cell tumors or tumors of low malignant potential. These tumor types exhibit a markedly more indolent course, and the metastatic behavior of these tumors is in direct apposition to the typical epithelial cell ovarian tumor for which screening programs are being designed. A PPV of 6% was reported in a more recent study in which 72 of 724 transvaginal ultrasounds were found to be abnormal, and the combination of transvaginal ultrasound and CA125 values achieved a PPV of 40% [28].

Combining CA125 and ultrasound screening modalities seems to be the most useful approach to screening high-risk patients; however, patients should be counseled about the limitations of screening alone.

Novel serum biomarkers have been identified and are being evaluated for use alone and in combination with CA125 for screening. Hellstrom et al. detected HE4 in the serum of patients with ovarian cancer with a greater sensitivity than CA125 (56.7% vs.10.8%) at the same specificity among the benign controls (100%) [34]. One trial examining multiple markers looked at the various combinations of nine markers including CA125, HE4, SMRP, CA72-4, osteopontin, ERBB2, inhibin, activin, and EGFR, and demonstrated that dual marker combination of CA125 and HE4 had a greater sensitivity than either marker alone [35]. Serum mesothelin was detected in 60% of ovarian cancer sera at 98% specificity. Importantly, mesothelin was shown to complement serum CA125 and the combination of the two markers detected a greater fraction of ovarian cancers than either marker alone [36]. Visintin et al. showed the combination of leptin, prolactin, osteopontin, insulin-like growth factor II, macrophage inhibitory factor, and CA-125 detected ovarian cancer with a specificity of 99.4% and sensitivity of 95.3% [37]. Preliminary data utilizing serum proteomics is also being evaluated for potential clinical utility, but has not yet been sufficiently validated for use in a prospective ovarian cancer screening trial [38].

Prevention of Ovarian Cancer in High-Risk Populations

Oral contraceptives (OCs) have been suggested as potential preventative agents that may reduce the subsequent risk of ovarian cancer [39–51]. Historically, the effect has been attributed to reduction in the number of ovulatory events with the regular use of OCs. More recent data, however, suggest the protective effect of OCs may be more complex. An innovative study examined the effect of ovarian epithelium of levonorgestrel in 130 ovulatory macaque monkeys, supporting the use of progestins as chemoprotective agents in ovarian cancer [39]. Levonorgestrel was administered over a period of 35 months, and the ovarian epithelium was examined for apoptosis using immunohistochemical techniques. Apoptotic cell counts in the ovarian epithelium were significantly increased in animals exposed to progesterone, and the authors hypothesized that progestin-induced apoptosis of the ovarian epithelium is responsible for the chemoprotective effect of OCs [39]. This hypothesis is a departure from the widely accepted theory that suppression of incessant ovulation is responsible for the reduced risk of ovarian cancer. The authors also theorized that OC progestins may decrease the risk of ovarian cancer by increasing the tendency of ovarian epithelial cells that have incurred genetic damage but are not yet neoplastic to undergo apoptotic death [40].

Several studies have suggested that the degree of protection is associated with the duration of use of OCs [45, 47, 48, 52–54]. The length of protection seems to be strongly correlated with duration of use. Prolonged risk reduction has been reported when OCs are used longer than 4–6 years, and minimal benefit has been observed if use is restricted to 6 months to 2 years [45, 47, 53, 54]. Furthermore, the protective benefit of OCs diminishes with time after discontinuing use and returns to baseline approximately 15 years after the last regular use of OCs [45, 47, 48].

The influence of the estrogen/progestin content of a particular OC on the subsequent ovarian cancer risk is an issue needing further study. Ness et al. demonstrated identical risk reduction for OCs with high-estrogen/high-progesterone content when compared with low estrogen/low-progesterone content pills [55]. More recently, low estrogen/low progestin OCs were found to significantly reduce the risk of ovarian carcinoma (odds ratio 0.19; 95% CI 0.05–0.75), and the risk was lower than among users of high potency OCs, but the difference was not statistically significant. Furthermore, an increased progesterone dose resulted in a significant increase in ovarian cancer risk, indicating a dose–response association [56].

One of the strongest risk factors for the development of ovarian cancer is a history of multiple affected family members. Studies by Gross et al. and Tavani et al. demonstrated a risk reduction with OC use in women with strong family histories [57, 58]. These results led Tavani et al. to suggest that 5 years of OC use in "high-risk women" can reduce ovarian cancer risk to the level observed in studies of low-risk women and in high-risk women who never used OCs but have parity as a protective factor [58]. Further study, however, of the association between OCs and ovarian cancer in *BRCA1* or *BRCA2* gene mutation carriers is needed. While an initial study of 207 women with confirmed *BRCA1/BRCA2* mutations demonstrated a statistically significant risk reduction with OC use, a reduction in the odds of ovarian cancer in women with *BRCA* mutations was reported to be only 0.2% per year of OC use (–4.9% to 5.0%) in a subsequent study [42, 59]. The protective effect of OCs would appear to be consistent across races as John et al. demonstrated a reduction risk of 0.6 in African-American women with OC use of 6 years or more [46].

Surgical Strategies to Reduce the Risk of Ovarian Cancer

Prophylactic surgical interventions are an option for patients who are at high risk of developing ovarian cancer. The effectiveness of risk reducing surgery in patients carrying *BRCA* gene mutations has been confirmed. Patients with *BRCA1* and *BRCA2* who undergo prophylactic bilateral salpingo-oophorectomy (BSO) reduce their risk of ovarian, fallopian tube, and peritoneal cancer by 80% [60]. A protective benefit for subsequent development of both breast and ovarian cancer in *BRCA* mutation-positive individuals undergoing risk reduction BSO has been observed in multiple studies [61, 62]. The hazard ratio for the development of breast cancer or *BRCA*-related gynecologic cancer after risk-reducing BSO was 0.25 (95% CI, 0.08–0.74) [62]. In order to reduce the risk, patients with *BRCA* mutations should consider prophylactic BSO around age 35 after the completion of childbearing [63]. Patients should be aware, however, that the survival benefit of undergoing prophylactic oophorectomy is minimal in women older than 60 [64].

A substantial number of women undergoing prophylactic oophorectomy will have an occult cancer of the ovaries identified on histological review. One study identified 11 cancers in 490 women at the time of prophylactic BSO with a prevalence of 2.4% in *BRCA1* and 1.8% in *BRCA2* mutation carriers undergoing the operation [64]. Rebbeck et al. found six stage I ovarian cancers among 259 *BRCA* mutation carriers at the time of procedure [61]. Occult ovarian, tubal, or peritoneal neoplasia was identified in 9.7% of women with known *BRCA1* and *BRCA2* mutations. Interestingly, many of the occult neoplasms identified using careful surgical and pathologic protocol occur in the fallopian tube at a rate of 52% [65].

Since many of the cancers identified at the time of prophylactic oophorectomy are microscopic, care must be taken to ensure removal of the entire ovaries and fallopian tubes. The surgical procedure should be performed by an experienced surgeon and serial sections of the specimens examined by an experienced pathologist. The surgeon should minimize the possibility of adhesions, endometriosis, and other inflammatory processes that predispose to the development of ovarian remnants. Cytologic evaluation is suggested, but not required as part of the procedure [63]. The fallopian tubes should be ligated as close to the uterine cornua as possible due to the high risk of malignant transformation [66]. Conflicting data exists over whether hysterectomy should be performed in addition to BSO in the context of risk-reduction surgery [67]. Currently, no conclusive evidence has been reported to support hysterectomy at the time of BSO.

Patients undergoing prophylactic oophorectomy must be counseled that the reduction in risk of ovarian and breast cancers is not absolute. One study reported that of 324 women who had undergone prophylactic oophorectomy, six women (2%) were identified who developed ovarian-type cancer, either from a remnant segment of ovarian tissue or carcinoma of the peritoneal cavity 27 years after surgery [68]. Rebbeck et al. identified 2 (0.8%) of 259 women with *BRCA* mutations who underwent prophylactic oophorectomy who were subsequently diagnosed with papillary serous peritoneal carcinoma 3.8 and 8.6 years after surgery, and breast cancer developed in 21 (21%) of 99 women who underwent prophylactic BSO [61]. In another study, subsequent breast cancer was diagnosed in 3 of 98 women who underwent prophylactic BSO during a mean follow-up of 24.2 months [62]. Although the risk of developing subsequent cancer after risk-reduction surgery is present, the overall risk reduction with prophylactic surgery warrants its use. The estimated proportion of women free from breast cancer or *BRCA*-related gynecologic cancer at 5 years was significantly greater in the group of patients who underwent prophylactic oophorectomy than the group who underwent surveillance, 94 and 69%, respectively [62]. Importance should be placed on continued close surveillance of patients after risk-reduction surgery is performed.

While not recommended as a sole procedure for prophylaxis against the development of ovarian cancer, retrospective reviews of women have noted a decreased risk of developing ovarian cancer among women following tubal ligation [42, 69–74]. This interesting finding suggests that limiting exposure of the ovary to environmental carcinogens may prevent the development of ovarian cancer. The ability of tubal ligation to reduce the risk of ovarian cancer appears to be operative in women with *BRCA1* and *BRCA2* mutations. One study compared 232 *BRCA*-positive women with a history of ovarian cancer to 232 *BRCA*-positive control women [71]. A history of tubal ligation was associated with a statistically significant reduction in risk by 63%. Despite the protective effect of tubal ligation, removal of the adjacent ovaries when laparoscopic surgery is contemplated in women at elevated risk due to genetic testing or strong family history of ovarian cancer is prudent.

Other Gynecological Malignancies Associated with Inherited Risk

Endometrial Carcinoma

Although endometrial carcinoma is the most common gynecological malignancy in the general population, it typically is not observed to be associated with elevated inherited risk in and of itself. However, in women who inherit HNPCC-associated germline mutations, an increased risk of endometrial cancer is observed. Endometrial cancer is the most frequent extracolonic cancer, and its cumulative lifetime risk has been estimated up to 60% [75]. The highest incidence for HNPCC-related endometrial cancer is between ages 40 and 60 [76]. More than 75% of the women with Lynch syndrome who develop endometrial cancer will present with stage 1 disease, and the 5-year survival rate is similar to that for sporadic endometrial cancer at 88% [77, 78]. A recent study by Walsh et al. recommends screening for HNPCC in any woman diagnosed with endometrial cancer prior to age 45 or synchronous endometrial and ovarian cancers, irrespective of family history [79].

Consideration of endometrial cancer screening in patients with Lynch syndrome is reasonable. The International Collaborative Group on Hereditary Nonpolyposis Colorectal Cancer recommends annual or biannual transvaginal ultrasound beginning at age 30–35 [80]. However, the efficacy of gynecologic screening procedures of patients with HNPCC-associated mutations has not been proven. Regular surveillance yielded no clinical benefit in a prospective trial with 269 females from HNPCC or HNPCC-like families. No asymptomatic cancer cases were found in 522 transvaginal ultrasound examinations but two interval cancers were diagnosed based on symptoms [81]. Annual endometrial biopsy beginning at age 30–35 has also been recommended for screening of women with HNPCC [82]. The combination of ultrasound and endometrial biopsy was shown to be fairly sensitive (82–98%) and specific in a study of symptomatic postmenopausal women, but its sensitivity in premenopausal women is uncertain [83]. All HNPCC-mutation carriers who are to undergo abdominal surgery for colorectal cancer must have a thorough gynecologic examination with endometrial biopsy preoperatively to exclude synchronous malignant or premalignant endometrial processes [80].

Prophylactic hysterectomy with BSO has been suggested as a reasonable management strategy for patients with HNPCC mutations. One study among women with documented germline mutations associated with HNPCC, no occurrences of endometrial, ovarian, or primary peritoneal cancers were reported in the 61 women who underwent prophylactic hysterectomy and the 47 women who underwent prophylactic BSO [84]. Therefore, in patients who have completed childbearing, prophylactic hysterectomy with BSO is a useful strategy for preventing endometrial and ovarian cancer associated with HNPCC.

Cervical Carcinoma

Gynecologic malignancies with increased inherited risk are exceedingly rare outside the scope of ovarian and endometrial cancer. Peutz–Jeghers syndrome is an autosomal dominant syndrome where individuals are prone to the development of intestinal polyps and subsequent malignancy of the gastrointestinal tract and pancreas. In addition to the association with ovarian sex cord stromal tumors with annular tubules as mentioned previously, women affected with this syndrome are also at increased risk for adenoma malignum or minimal deviation adenocarcinoma (MDC) of the cervix [85, 86].

Histologically, MDC is characterized by cytologically bland glands that penetrate the cervical stroma to a depth not typically encountered. Due to the deep involvement of the glands, a cone biopsy is often indicated in the diagnostic management of this disorder. When diagnosed, the treatment of MDC is radical hysterectomy, while radiation therapy is preferred in more advanced stage disease.

Conclusion

A careful personal and family history of cancer can identify those who would benefit from screening and potential genetic testing. The ideal candidates for genetic testing are those patients affected by breast and/or ovarian cancer. If a specific mutation is identified, other family members can be tested for that specific mutation, making the test more affordable. Patients must be counseled that a negative test in a high-risk family may be secondary to a current unidentified mutation and not evidence that they are not at risk. Limitations to current screening methods warrant further study to identify the best screening modalities for ovarian cancer. The OCs have a protective effect independent of race or risk, but details on the length of use and specific combination used have yet to be determined. Prophylactic surgery appears to be beneficial for patients with *BRCA1* and *BRCA2* mutations, as well as patients with HNPCC mutations.

References

1. Easton D, Ford D, Bishop D. Breast Cancer Linkage Consortium: Breast and ovarian cancer incidence in *BRCA1* mutation carriers. Am J Hum Genet 1995;56:265–271.
2. Beller U, Halle D, Catane R, et al. High frequency of *BRCA1* and *BRCA2* gene mutations in Ashkenazi Jewish ovarian cancer patients, regardless of family history. Gynecol Oncol 1997;67:123–126.
3. Antoniou A, Pharoah PDP, Narod S, et al. Average risk of breast and ovarian cancer associated with *BRCA1* or *BRCA2* mutations detected in case series unselected for family history: A combined analysis of 22 studies. Am J Hum Genet 2003;72:1117–1130.
4. Ford D, Easton D, Stratton M, et al. Genetic heterogeneity and penetrance analysis of the *BRCA1* and *BRCA2* genes in breast cancer families. Am J Hum Genet 1998;62:676–689.
5. Gayther S, Russell R, Harrington P, et al. The contribution of germline *BRCA1* and *BRCA2* mutations to familial ovarian cancer: No evidence for other ovarian cancer susceptibility genes. Am J Hum Genet 1999;65:1021–1029.
6. Lallas T, Beukers T, Buller R. *BRCA1* mutations in familial ovarian cancer. Mol Genet Met 1999;67:357–363.
7. Reddy M, Gallion H, Fowler J, et al. Contribution of *BRCA1* and *BRCA2* to familial ovarian cancer: A Gynecology Oncology Group study. Gynecol Oncol 2002;85:255–259.
8. Sutcliffe S, Pharoah P, Easton D, et al. Ovarian and breast cancer risk to women in families with two or more cases of ovarian cancer. Int J Cancer 2000;87:110–117.
9. Welcsh P, Owens K, King M. Insights into the functions of *BRCA1* and *BRCA2*. Trends Genet 2000;16:69–74.
10. Tutt A and Ashworth A. The relationship between the roles of *BRCA* genes in DNA repair and cancer predisposition. Trends Mol Med 2002;8:571–576.
11. Sharan SK, Morimatsu M, Albrecht U, et al. Embryonic lethality and radiation hypersensitivity mediated by Rad51 in mice lacking *BRCA2*. Nature 1999;386:804–810.

12. Scully R, Chen J, Plug A, et al. Association of *BRCA1* with Rad51 in mitotic and meiotic cells. Cell 1997;88:265–275.
13. Sowter HM and Ashworth A. *BRCA1* and *BRCA2* as ovarian cancer susceptibility genes. Carcinogenesis 2005;26:1651–1656.
14. Stratton J, Gayther S, Russell P, et al. Contribution of *BRCA1* mutations to ovarian cancer. N Engl J Med 1997;336:1125–1130.
15. Lynch H and de la Chapelle A. Hereditary colorectal cancer. N Engl J Med 2003;348:919–932.
16. South S, Vance H, Farrell C, et al. Consideration of hereditary nonpolyposis colorectal cancer in *BRCA* mutation-negative familial ovarian cancers. Cancer 2009;115:324–333.
17. Malander S, Rambech E, Kristoffersson U, et al. The contribution of the hereditary nonpolyposis colorectal cancer syndrome to the development of ovarian cancer. Gynecol Oncol 2006;101:238–243.
18. Shaw P, McLaughlin J, Zweemer R, et al. Histopathologic features of genetically determined ovarian cancer. Int J Gynecol Pathol 2002;21:407–411.
19. Young R, Dickersin G, Scully R. Juvenile granulosa cell tumor of the ovary: A clinicopathological analysis of 125 cases. Am J Surg Pathol 1984;8:575–596.
20. Hartmann L, Young R, Evans M, Podratz K. Ovarian sex cord-stromal. In: Hoskins W, Perez C, Young R, eds. Principles and Practice of Gynecologic Oncology. 2nd ed. Philadelphia: Lippincott-Raven; 1997:1013–1015.
21. Raggio M, Kaplan A, Harberg J. Recurrent ovarian fibromas with basal cell nevus syndrome (Gorlin syndrome). Obstet Gynecol 1983;61:95–97.
22. Narita T, Takagi K. Ataxia telangiectasia with dysgerminoma of the right ovary, papillary carcinoma of the thyroid and adenocarcinoma of the pancreas. Cancer 1984;54:113–116.
23. Troche V, Hernandez E. Neoplasia arising in dysgentic gonads. Obstet Gynecol Surv 1986;41:74–79.
24. The NCCN Genetic/Familial High-Risk Assessment: Breast and Ovarian Clinical Practice Guidelines in Oncology (Version 1.2009). © 2009 National Comprehensive Cancer Network, Inc. Available at: http://www.nccn.org. Accessed January 30, 2010.
25. Palma M, Ristori E, Ricevuto E, et al. *BRCA1* and *BRCA2*: The genetic testing and the current management options for mutation carriers. Crit Rev Oncol Hemat 2006;57:1–23.
26. NIH Consensus Development Panel on Ovarian Cancer. Ovarian Cancer: Screening, treatment, and follow-up. JAMA 1995;273:491–497.
27. Jacobs I, Davies AP, Bridges J, et al. Prevalence screening for ovarian cancer in postmenopausal women by CA125 measurement and ultrasonography. Br Med J 1993;306:1030–1034.
28. Olivier RI, Lubsen-Brandsma MAC, Verhoef S, and van Beurden M. CA125 and transvaginal ultrasound monitoring in high-risk women cannot prevent the diagnosis of advanced ovarian cancer. Gynecol Oncol 2006;100:20–26.
29. Einhorn N, Sjovall K, Knapp RC, et al. Prospective evaluation of serum CA125 levels for early detection of ovarian cancer. Obstet Gynecol 1992;80:14–18.
30. Skates SJ, Xu FJ, Yu YH, et al. Toward an optimal algorithm for ovarian cancer screening with longitudinal tumor markers. Cancer 1995;76:2004–2010.
31. Menon U, Skates S, Lewis S, et al. Prospective study using the risk of ovarian cancer algorithm to screen for ovarian cancer. J Clin Oncol 2005;23:7919–7926.
32. Van Nagell JR Jr, DePriest PD, Reedy MB, et al. The efficacy of transvaginal sonographic screening in asymptomatic women at risk of ovarian cancer [see comments]. Gynecol Oncol 2000;77:350–356.
33. Sato S, Yokoyama Y, Sakamoto T, et al. Usefulness of mass screening for ovarian carcinoma using transvaginal ultrasonography. Cancer 2000;89:582–588.
34. Hellstrom I, Raycraft J, Hayden-Ledbetter M, et al. The HE4 (WFDC2) protein is a biomarker for ovarian carcinoma. Cancer Res 2003;63:3695–3700.
35. Moore A, Brown M, Miller S, et al. The use of multiple novel tumor biomarkers for the detection of ovarian carcinoma in patients with a pelvic mass. Gynecol Oncol 2007;108:402–408.
36. McIntosh M, Drescher C, Karlan B, et al. Combining CA125 and SMR serum markers for diagnosis and early detection of ovarian carcinoma. Gynecol Oncol 2004;95:9–15.

37. Visintin I, Feng Z, Longton G, et al. Diagnostic markers for early detection of ovarian cancer. Clin Cancer Res 2008;14:1065–1072.
38. Rosenthal AN, Menon U, Jacobs IJ. Screening for ovarian cancer. Clin Obstet Gynecol 2006;49:433–447.
39. Rodriguez GC, Walmer DK, Cline M, et al. Effect of progestin on the ovarian epithelium of macaques: Cancer prevention through apoptosis? J Soc Gynecol Invest 1998;5:271–276.
40. Ness RB, Grisso JA, Vergona R, et al. Oral contraceptives, other methods of contraception, and risk reduction for ovarian cancer. Epidemiology 2001;12:307–312.
41. Siskind V, Green A, Bain C, et al. Beyond ovulation: Oral contraceptives and epithelial ovarian cancer. Epidemiology 2000;11:106–110.
42. Narod SA, Risch H, Moslehi R, et al. Oral contraceptives and the risk of hereditary ovarian cancer. Hereditary Ovarian Cancer Clinical Study Group. N Engl J Med 1998;339:424–428.
43. Vessey MP, Painter R. Endometrial and ovarian cancer and oral contraceptives-findings in a large cohort study. Br J Cancer 1995;71:1340–1342.
44. Hankinson SE, Colditz GA, Hunter DJ, et al. A prospective study of reproductive factors and risk of epithelial ovarian cancer. Cancer 1995;76:284–290.
45. Rosenberg L, Palmer JR, Zauber AG, et al. A case-control study of oral contraceptive use and invasive epithelial ovarian cancer. Am J Epidemiol 1994;139:654–661.
46. John EM, Whittemore AS, Harris R, et al. Characteristics relating to ovarian cancer risk: Collaborative analysis of seven US case control studies. Epithelial ovarian cancer in black women. Collaborative Ovarian Cancer Group. JNCI 1993;85:142–147.
47. Parazzini F, La Vechia C, Negri E, et al. Oral contraceptive use and the risk of ovarian cancer: An Italian case control study. Eur J Cancer 1991;27:594–598.
48. Franceschi S, Parazzini F, Negri E, et al. Pooled analysis of 3 European case-control studies of epithelial ovarian cancer. Oral contraceptive use. Int J Cancer 1991;49:61–65.
49. Parazzini F, Restelli C, La Vechia C, et al. Risk factors for epithelial ovarian tumors of borderline malignancy. Int J Epidemiol 1991;20:871–877.
50. Gwinn ML, Lee NC, Rhodes PH. Pregnancy, breast feeding, and oral contraceptives and the risk of epithelial ovarian cancer. J Clin Epidemiol 1990;43:559–568.
51. The Cancer and Steroid Hormone Study of the Centers for Disease Control and the National Institute of Child Health and Human Development. The reduction of risk of ovarian cancer associated with oral contraceptive use. N Engl J Med 1987;316:650–655.
52. Wu ML, Whittemore AS, Paffenbarger RS Jr, et al. Personal and environmental characteristics related to epithelial ovarian cancer: Reproductive and menstrual events and oral contraceptive use. Am J Epidemiol 1988;128:1216–1227.
53. Gross TP, Schlesselman JJ, Stadel BV, et al. The risk of epithelial ovarian cancer in short-term users of oral contraceptives. Am J Epidemiol 1992;136:46–53.
54. Hartge P, Whittemore A, Itnyre J, et al. Rates and risk of ovarian cancer in subgroups of white women in the United States. The Collaborative Ovarian Cancer Group. Obstet Gynecol 1994;84:760–764.
55. Ness RB, Grisso JA, Klapper J, et al. Risk of ovarian cancer in relation to estrogen and progestin dose and use characteristics of oral contraceptives. SHARE Study Group. Steroid hormones and reproductions. Am J Epidemiol 2000;152:233–241.
56. Lurie G, Thompson P, McDuffie KE, et al. Association of estrogen and progestin potency of oral contraceptives with ovarian carcinoma risk. Obstet Gynecol 2007;109:597–607.
57. Gross TP, Schlesselman JJ. The estimated effect of oral contraceptive use on the cumulative risk of ovarian cancer. Obstet Gynecol 1994;83:419–424.
58. Tavani A, Ricci E, La Vechia C, et al. Influence of menstrual and reproductive factors on ovarian cancer risk in women with and without family history of breast or ovarian cancer. Int J Epidemiol 2000;29:799–802.
59. Modan B, Hartge P, Hirsh-Yechezkel G, et al. Parity, oral contraceptives, and the risk of ovarian cancer among carriers and noncarriers of BRCA1 or BRCA2 mutation. N Engl J Med 2001;345:235–240.

60. Finch A, Beiner M, Lubinski J, et al. Salpingo-oophorectomy and the risk of ovarian, fallopian tube, and peritoneal cancers in women with *BRCA1* or *BRCA2* mutations. JAMA 2006;296:185–192.
61. Rebbeck TR, Lynch HT, Neuhausen SL, et al. Prophylactic oophorectomy in carriers of *BRCA1* or *BRCA2* mutations. N Engl J Med 2002;346:1616–1622.
62. Kauff ND, Satagopan JM, Robson M, et al. Risk-reducing salpingo-oophorectomy in women with a *BRCA1* or *BRCA2* mutation. N Engl J Med 2002;346:1609–1615.
63. SGO Committee Statement. Society of Gynecologic Oncologists Clinical Practice Committee Statement on Prophylactic Salpingo-oophorectomy. Gynecol Oncol 2005;98:179–181.
64. Schrag D, Kuntz KM, Garber JE, et al. Decision analysis-effects of prophylactic mastectomy and oophorectomy on life expectancy among women with *BRCA1* or *BRCA2* mutations. N Engl J Med 1997;336:1465–1471.
65. Lamb JD, Garcia RL, Goff BA, et al. Predictors of occult neoplasia in women undergoing risk-reducing salpingo-oophorectomy. Am J Obstet Gynecol 2006;194:1702–1709.
66. Aziz S, Kuperstein G, Rose B, et al. A genetic epidemiological study of carcinoma of the fallopian tube. Gynecol Oncol 2001;80:341–345.
67. Karlan BY. Defining cancer risks for *BRCA* germline mutation carriers: Implications for surgical prophylaxis. Gynecol Oncol 2004;92:519–520.
68. Piver MS, Jishi MF, Tsukada Y, et al. Primary peritoneal carcinoma after prophylactic oophorectomy in women with a family history of ovarian cancer: A report of the Gilda Radner Familial Ovarian Cancer Registry. Cancer 1993;71:2751–2755.
69. Cornelison T, Natarajan N, Piver M, et al. Tubal ligation and the risk of ovarian carcinoma. Cancer Detect Prev 1997;21:1–6.
70. Hankinson S, Hunter D, Colditz G, et al. Tubal ligation, hysterectomy, and risk of ovarian cancer. A prospective study. JAMA 1993;270:2813–2818.
71. Narod SA, Sun P, Ghadirian P, et al. Tubal ligation and risk of ovarian cancer in carriers of *BRCA1* or *BRCA2* mutations: A case-control study. Lancet 2001;357:1467–1470.
72. Miracle-McMahill HL, Calle EE, Kosinski AS, et al. Tubal ligation and fatal ovarian cancer in a larger prospective cohort study. Am J Epidemiol 1997;14:349–357.
73. Green A, Purdie D, Bain C, et al. Tubal sterilization, hysterectomy and decreased risk of ovarian cancer: Survey of women's health study group. Int J Cancer 1997;71:948–951.
74. Rosenblatt KA and Thomas DB. Reduced risk of ovarian cancer in women with a tubal ligation or hysterectomy: The World Health Organization collaborative study of neoplasia and steroid contraceptives. Cancer Epidemiol Biomarkers Prev 1996;5:933–935.
75. Aarnio M, Sankila R, Pukkala E, et al. Cancer risk in mutation carriers of DNA-mismatch-repair genes. Int J Cancer 1999;81:214–218.
76. Watson P, Vasen HFA, Mecklin JP, et al. The risk of endometrial cancer in hereditary nonpolyposis colorectal cancer. Am J Med 1994;96:516–520.
77. Broaddus RR, Lynch HT, Chen LM, et al. Pathologic features of endometrial carcinoma associated with HNPCC. Cancer 2006;106:87–94.
78. Boks DE, Trujillo AP, Voogd AC, et al. Survival analysis of endometrial carcinoma associated with hereditary nonpolyposis colorectal cancer. Int J Cancer 2002;102:198–200.
79. Walsh C, Blum A, Walts A, et al. Lynch syndrome among gynecology patients meeting Bethesda guidelines for screening. Gynecol Oncol 2009;doi:10.1016/j.gyno. 2009.11.021.
80. Abdel-Rahman WM, Mecklin JP, Peltomaki P. The genetics of HNPCC: Application to diagnosis and screening. Crit Rev Oncol Hematol 2006;58:208–220.
81. Dove-Edwin I, Boks D, Goff S, et al. The outcome of endometrial carcinoma surveillance by ultrasound scan in women at risk of hereditary nonpolyposis colorectal carcinoma and familial colorectal carcinoma. Cancer 2002;94:1708–1712.
82. Lindor LM, Peterson GM, Hadley DW, et al. Recommendations for the care of individuals with an inherited predisposition to Lynch syndrome: A systematic review. JAMA 2009;296:1507–1517.
83. Van den Bosch T, Van den Dael A, Van Schouboreck D, et al. Combining vaginal ultrasonography and office endometrial sampling in the diagnosis of endometrial disease in postmenopausal women. Obstet Gynecol 1995;85:349–352.

84. Schmeler KM, Lynch HT, Chen L, et al. Prophylactic surgery to reduce the risk of gynecologic cancers in the Lynch syndrome. N Engl J Med 2006;354:261–269.
85. Gilks C, Young R, Aguirre P, et al. Adenoma malignum (minimal deviation adenocarcinoma) of the uterine cervix: A clinicopathological and immunohistochemical analysis of 26 cases. Am J Surg Pathol 1989;13:707–714.
86. Kaminsky P and Norris H. Minimal deviation carcinoma (adenoma malignum) of the cervix. Int J Gynecol Pathol 1983;12:141–145.

Index